# Message
With Love

To

## All, Present and Future Generations

And Thanks To
Patent-Lawyer Ohriner, Members of Congress Norton and Van Hollen

# Contents

# Acknowledgment

Author is grateful to the experts named for help in art,
review and edit the Book.


Cover page/Illustrations:
Bot Roda, Artist


Editor/Reviewer:
Anna Scrimenti          Edit & Review
Raghava Rao Mandava          Review

# Preface

## Why Sleep Method—Why Not Pills?

The ability to breathe, eat, and sleep comes with birth and is essential to sustain life. Thus sleep is essential for the survival of life.

The method to induce instant sleep describes a simple process that will help activate the brain and produce melatonin to invite sleep and serotonin to make the brain fall asleep at any time—day or night—when a person wants to sleep. This process doesn't require the user to take sleeping pills or drugs which could adversely affect the health, perhaps shortening life or causing cancer.

It is a simple process that one can learn, practice, and master for beneficial use. The simple devices described aid the user in practicing this method. Primarily, the method involves two steps: the first step is to calm the mind from intrusive thoughts; and the second step is to split the two hemispheres of the brain and stop them from communicating with each other. At the instant when the two hemispheres stop communicating, the brain falls asleep. This two-step process frees the mind from stress, anxiety, anger, and depression and puts the brain into a sleep cycle.

The skill learned through proper use of the process described here can improve a person's ability to breathe properly and sleep well for a healthy and happy life. The author had to spend 10 percent of his life time—with a life after Leukemia, to obtain patent protection. See the Appendix if interested to learn more about it. Or if your interest is primarily to learn the 'method' quickly, skip the Appendix and other details, and go directly to Figures 3.5-3.9 and Chapter 5, and review the material carefully. Place an order for the devices, and go to practice the method on your own upon receiving the devices. You can also enroll into a class near you to learn the process, if required. To find out more on the benefit of a good night sleep, please see the introduction to the study on wake-sleep state of the brain.

Good Luck!

The Author

# Introduction

Research *news* on Wake-Sleep state of the Brain

**From:** Mikki
**Sent:** Sunday, October 20, 2013 7:53 AM
**To:** 'health-science@washpost.com'
**Cc:** 'nedergaard@urmc.rochester.edu'; lars.heikensten@nobel.se; 'sjensen@ Waisman.Wisc.Edu'; 'wagner@emory.edu'; overbye@nytimes.com
**Subject:** 'Brains flush toxic waste in sleep, including Alzheimer's-linked protein- study of mice finds

10/20/13

Dear Meeri:

Good research and good article. I wrote to the researcher already. See a copy of my message to Dr. Nedergaard sent couple of days back.

However, if she insists on putting 'pills' or 'drugs' into the brain "to force a cleanup"- she is mistaken- that might give some temporary relief to the brain-disease, but would hasten death of the brain.

Please read my Book: 'Induce Instant sleep' (will be available by end of this month thru Amazon.com, Books)- that is the tool or skill required to cure most of the common Brain-diseases.

By the way, a few years ago, MRI studies were conducted by Prof. Davidson at the U of Wisconsin with the help of Dalai Lama Monks:

The brain activity of the Monks were observed and recorded when awake and when under deep meditation. Please see an old article in Washington Post (attached below).

The MRI results show similar activity as in the present study at U of Rochester. So, these two studies deserve a Nobel (not like the one in the case of fake 'god particle').
Maheswar

---

**From:** Mikki

Friday, October 18, 2013 9:27 AM
**To:** 'nedergaard@urmc.rochester.edu'
**Cc:** lars.heikensten@nobel.se;...
**Subject:** Sleep

10/18/13

Dear Prof. Nedergaard:

I read an MSNBC news article below regarding your research on brain- wake-sleep state. I think and I know your findings are 'fundamental' in nature. If anyone deserves a Nobel for fundamental discovery in Neuroscience, this must be it. Thanks for your good work.

The cure for all or almost all brain diseases would be "sleep", not chemicals or pills.

I re-discovered a "method", an ancient-method that can make the brain 'fall asleep instantly' at any time one practices the method.

After a long struggle, recently I received a 'patent' for the method.

I wrote a Book: 'Induce Instant Sleep' which is being published (will be available in couple of weeks from now thru Amazon.com, Books). Please look into that and get back with me?

Please keep in touch.

Maheswar

---

## Study I:  University of Wisconsin

## Meditation Gives Brain a Charge, Study Finds: By Marc
Kaufman Washington Post Staff Writer
Monday, January 3, 2005

Brain research is beginning to produce concrete evidence for something that Buddhist practitioners of meditation have maintained for centuries: Mental discipline and meditative practice can change the workings of the brain and allow people to achieve different levels of awareness.

Those transformed states have traditionally been understood in transcendent terms, as something outside the world of physical measurement and objective evaluation. But over the past few years, researchers at the University of Wisconsin working with Tibetan monks have been able to translate those mental experiences into the scientific language of high-frequency gamma waves and brain synchrony, or coordination. And they have pinpointed the left prefrontal cortex, an area just behind the left forehead, as the place where brain activity associated with meditation is especially intense.

"What we found is that the longtime practitioners showed brain activation on a scale we have never seen before," said Richard Davidson, a neuroscientist at the university's new $10 million W.M. Keck Laboratory for Functional Brain Imaging and Behavior. "Their mental practice is having an effect on the brain in the same way golf or tennis practice will enhance performance." It demonstrates, he said, that the brain is capable of being trained and physically modified in ways few people can imagine.

Scientists used to believe the opposite -- that connections among brain nerve cells were fixed early in life and did not change in adulthood. But that assumption was disproved over the past decade with the help of advances in brain imaging and other techniques, and in its place, scientists have embraced the concept of ongoing brain development and "neuroplasticity."

Davidson says his newest results from the meditation study, published in the Proceedings of the National Academy of Sciences in November, take the concept of neuroplasticity a step further by showing that mental training through meditation (and presumably other disciplines) can itself change the inner workings and circuitry of the brain.

The new findings are the result of a long, if unlikely, collaboration between Davidson and Tibet's Dalai Lama, the world's best-known practitioner of Buddhism. The Dalai Lama first invited Davidson to his home in Dharamsala, India, in 1992 after learning about Davidson's innovative research into the neuroscience of emotions. The Tibetans have a centuries-old tradition of intensive meditation and, from the start, the Dalai Lama was interested in having Davidson scientifically explore the workings of his monks' meditating minds. Three years ago, the Dalai Lama spent two days visiting Davidson's lab.

The Dalai Lama ultimately dispatched eight of his most accomplished practitioners to Davidson's lab to have them hooked up for electroencephalograph (EEG) testing and brain scanning. The Buddhist practitioners in the experiment had undergone training in the Tibetan Nyingmapa and Kagyupa traditions of meditation for an estimated 10,000 to 50,000 hours, over time periods of 15 to 40 years. As a control, 10 student volunteers with no previous meditation experience were also tested after one week of training.

The monks and volunteers were fitted with a net of 256 electrical sensors and asked to meditate for short periods. Thinking and other mental activity are known to produce slight, but detectable, bursts of electrical activity as large groupings of neurons send messages to each other, and that's what the sensors picked up. Davidson was especially interested in measuring gamma waves, some of the highest-frequency and most important electrical brain impulses.

Both groups were asked to meditate, specifically on unconditional compassion. Buddhist teaching describes that state, which is at the heart of the Dalai Lama's teaching, as the "unrestricted readiness and availability to help living beings." The researchers chose that focus because it does not require concentrating on particular objects, memories or images, and cultivates instead a transformed state of being.

Davidson said that the results unambiguously showed that meditation activated the trained minds of the monks in significantly different ways from those of the volunteers. Most important, the electrodes picked up much greater activation of fast-moving and unusually powerful gamma waves in the monks, and found that the movement of the waves through the brain was far better organized and coordinated than in the students. The meditation novices showed only a slight increase in gamma wave activity while meditating, but some of the monks produced gamma wave activity more powerful than any previously reported in a healthy person, Davidson said.

The monks who had spent the most years meditating had the highest levels of gamma waves, he added. This "dose response" -- where higher levels of a drug or activity have greater effect than lower levels -- is what researchers look for to assess cause and effect.

In previous studies, mental activities such as focus, memory, learning and consciousness were associated with the kind of enhanced neural coordination found in the monks. The intense gamma waves found in the monks have also been associated with knitting together disparate brain circuits, and so are connected to higher mental activity and heightened awareness, as well.

Davidson's research is consistent with his earlier work that pinpointed the left prefrontal cortex as a brain region associated with happiness and positive thoughts and emotions. Using functional magnetic resonance imagining (fMRI) on the meditating monks, Davidson found that their brain activity -- as measured by the EEG -- was especially high in this area.

Davidson concludes from the research that meditation not only changes the workings of the brain in the short term, but also quite possibly produces permanent changes. That finding, he said, is based on the fact that the monks had considerably more gamma wave activity than the control group even before they started meditating. A researcher at the University of Massachusetts, Jon Kabat-Zinn, came to a similar conclusion several years ago.

Researchers at Harvard and Princeton universities are now testing some of the same monks on different aspects of their meditation practice: their ability to visualize images and control their thinking. Davidson is also planning further research.

"What we found is that the trained mind, or brain, is physically different from the untrained one," he said. In time, "we'll be able to better understand the potential importance of this kind of mental training and increase the likelihood that it will be taken seriously."

## Study II: University of Rochester

Brains flush toxic waste in sleep, including Alzheimer's-linked protein, study of mice finds: *By Meeri Kim,*

Washington Post, Published: October 19, 2013

While we are asleep, our bodies may be resting, but our brains are busy taking out the trash.

A new study has found that the cleanup system in the brain, responsible for flushing out toxic waste products that cells produce with daily use, goes into overdrive in mice that are asleep. The cells even shrink in size to make for easier cleaning of the spaces around them.

Study pinpoints another reason for sleep: to flush out toxic waste, including Alzheimer's-linked proteins.

Scientists say this nightly self-clean by the brain provides a compelling biological reason for the restorative power of sleep.

"Sleep puts the brain in another state where we clean out all the byproducts of activity during the daytime," said study author and University of Rochester neurosurgeon Maiken Nedergaard. Those byproducts include beta-amyloid protein, clumps of which form plaques found in the brains of Alzheimer's patients.

Staying up all night could prevent the brain from getting rid of these toxins as efficiently, and explain why sleep deprivation has such strong and immediate consequences. Too little sleep causes mental fog, crankiness, and increased risks of migraine and seizure. Rats deprived of all sleep die within weeks.

Although as essential and universal to the animal kingdom as air and water, sleep is a riddle that has baffled scientists and philosophers for centuries. Drifting off into a reduced consciousness seems evolutionarily foolish, particularly for those creatures in danger of getting eaten or attacked.

One line of thinking was that sleep helps animals to conserve energy by forcing a period of rest. But this theory seems unlikely since the sleeping brain uses up almost as much energy as the awake brain, Nedergaard said.

Another puzzle involves why different animals require different amounts of sleep per night. For instance, cats sleep more than 12 hours a day, while elephants need only about three hours. Based on this newfound purpose of sleep, neuroscientist Suzana Herculano-Houzel speculates in a commentary that the varying sleep needs across species might be related to brain size. Larger brains should have a relatively larger volume of space between cells, and may need less time to clean since they have more room for waste to accumulate throughout the day.

Sleep does play a key role in memory formation — mentally going through the events of the day and stamping certain memories into the brain. But sleeping for eight hours or more just to consolidate memories seems excessive, Nedergaard said, especially for an animal such as a mouse.

Last year, Nedergaard and her colleagues discovered a network that drains waste from the brain, which they dubbed the glymphatic system. It works by circulating cerebrospinal fluid throughout the brain tissue and flushing any resulting waste into the bloodstream, which then carries it to the liver for detoxification.

She then became curious about how the glymphatic system behaves during the sleep-wake cycle.

An imaging technique called two-photon microscopy enabled the scientists to watch the movement of cerebrospinal fluid through a live mouse brain in real time. After soothing the creature until it was sound asleep, study author Lulu Xie tagged the fluid with a special fluorescent dye.

"During sleep, the cerebrospinal fluid flushed through the brain very quickly and broadly," said Rochester neuropharmacologist Xie. As another experiment revealed, sleep causes the space between cells to increase by 60 percent, allowing the flow to increase.

Xie then gently touched the mouse's tail until it woke up from its nap, and she again injected it with dye. This time, with the mouse awake, flow in the brain was greatly constrained.

"Brain cells shrink when we sleep, allowing fluid to enter and flush out the brain," Nedergaard said. "It's like opening and closing a faucet."

They also found that the harmful beta-amyloid protein clears out of the brain twice as fast in a sleeping rodent as in an up-and-about one. The study was published in the journal Science on Thursday.

New York University cell biologist and Alzheimer's specialist Ralph A. Nixon, who was not involved in the study, said the findings could be of great interest to the Alzheimer's research community. For instance, the overproduction of beta-amyloid could be linked to the development of the disease, but he said these new findings hint that the lack of clearing it out might be the bigger problem.

Other neurodegenerative disorders, such as Parkinson's disease or chronic traumatic encephalopathy, are also associated with a backup of too much cell waste in the brain. "Clearance mechanisms may be very relevant to keeping these proteins at a level that isn't disease-causing," Nixon said.

An MRI diagnostic test for glymphatic clearance is in the works by Nedergaard and her colleagues. She also believes that a drug could be developed to force a cleanup if necessary, perhaps by mimicking the sleep-wake cycle.

*Meeri Kim is a freelance science journalist based in Philadelphia.*

# University of Rochester

## A good night's sleep scrubs your brain clean, research finds:

*By Barbara Mantel, NBC News contributor*

New research finds that a newly discovered system that flushes waste from your brain is mostly active during sleep.

It's no secret that too little shut-eye can drain your brain, but scientists haven't fully understood why.

Now, a new study suggests that a good night's sleep leaves you feeling sharp and refreshed because a newly discovered system that scrubs away neural waste is mostly active when you're at rest.

It's a revelation that could not only transform scientists' fundamental understanding of sleep, but also point to new ways to treat disorders such as Alzheimer's disease, which are linked to the accumulation of toxins in the brain.

"We have a cleaning system that almost stops when we are awake and starts when we sleep. It's almost like opening and closing a faucet -- it's that dramatic," says Dr. Maiken Nedergaard, co-director of the Center for Translational Neuromedicine at the University of Rochester Medical Center.

Nedergaard is the lead author of the study published Thursday in the journal Science. She and her colleagues first reported last year their discovery of the brain's unique waste removal system, dubbed the glymphatic system. It works like a neural trash truck, clearing away toxic by-products that build up when you're awake. The scientists had used two-photon microscopy — a new imaging technology that allows scientists to see deep inside living tissue — to peer into the brains of mice, which are remarkably similar to human brains.

They found that the glymphatic system pumps cerebral spinal fluid, CSF, through the spaces around the brain cells, flushing waste into the circulatory system, where it eventually makes its way to the liver.

Their latest research, also in mice, used the same technology to focus on the timing of the glymphatic system. The researchers discovered that during sleep brain cells contract, increasing the space between the cells by as much as 60 percent and allowing the spinal fluid to wash more freely through the brain tissue.

"This study shows that the brain has different functional states when asleep and when awake," Nedergaard says. "In fact, the restorative nature of sleep appears to be the result of the active clearance of the by-products of neural activity that accumulate during wakefulness."

The scientists found that the glymphatic system was almost 10 times more active during sleep than when awake.

"The brain has only limited energy at its disposal and it appears that it must choose between two different functional states — awake and aware or asleep and cleaning up," Nedergaard said. "You can think of it like having a house party. You can either entertain guests or clean up the house, but you can't really do both at the same time."

One of the waste products of the brain is the protein amyloid-beta, which accumulates and forms plaques in the brains of Alzheimer's patients. Researchers at Washington University in St. Louis had previously shown that levels of amyloid-beta in mice brains dropped during sleep because of a decrease in production of the protein.

"That was an observation that inspired our work," says Nedergaard, "and we decided to look at clearance."

Both lower production of amyloid-beta and faster clearance are likely key to lower levels of amyloid-beta during sleep, says Nedergaard. Her view is echoed by Dr. Yo-El Ju, a professor of neurology and a member of Washington University's research team.

"Possibly there are both mechanisms working that produce the large variations between wake and sleep that we see," says Ju.

Patients with diseases that cause progressive brain decline — Alzheimer's, Parkinson's and Lewy Body dementia — often sleep poorly. The diseases are also associated with the abnormal buildup of protein in the brain.

While researchers don't yet know if these plaques are a cause or a result of neurodegenerative disease, the new insights about the way sleep clears waste from the brain could lead to new treatment approaches, according to both Ju and Nedergaard.

"In addition to trying to decrease the amount of amyloid-beta production, perhaps we can also try to increase the amount of clearance," says Ju.

Nedergaard and colleagues are testing possible drugs in mice that could do that.

"Understanding how and when the brain activates the glymphatic system and clears waste is a critical first step in efforts to potentially modulate the system and make it work more efficiently," Nedergaard says.

Research in humans has shown that levels of amyloid-beta decline during sleep, as it does in mice, but it's not yet known if the mechanisms are the same as in mice.

"Those experiments in humans to measure both production and clearance during wake and sleep are ongoing. We don't have the results yet," says Ju.

*JoNel Aleccia of NBC News contributed to this report.*

# Chapter: 1

## Begin the Process

Adam, the teacher, walks into a conference room with sofas and beds set out; the room is filled with pupils wanting to learn the process that induces instant sleep. The staff member who organized the class welcomes the teacher, introduces him to the class, and requests, "Please sit down in a sofa or on a bed wherever you feel comfortable. Now, our teacher will begin to teach the process."

One of the waiting pupils gets up, walks closer to the teacher, and introduces herself: I am Eve. I have come here to meet with you—I am not sure if anyone can help me with my problem.

Adam:
Are not you the singer and dancer I have seen on TV—the famous artist the world has known?

Eve:
Maybe you have seen me as a singer and dancer, not as a sleepless drug addict. I am here seeking your help. I can't fall asleep without taking a fistful of pills every night. That makes me sick and tired the next morning. That's my problem. Can you help me?

Adam:
Yes, I can give it a try. I can only teach you the method. The rest is in your own hands. You need to practice and practice until you become a master in the skill of inducing sleep, like you practiced the art of singing and dancing as if it were a second nature. I am sure you can do it, but only if you are ready to put your mind to it. This method works whether you are under great stress or anxiety or even depressed for any reason, including bodily ailments such as aches and pains. In fact, you do not necessarily have to have a problem in falling asleep

to learn this method. The method comes in handy whenever one wants to take a nap or fall asleep for an hour or more to be fresh and energetic. And, one can fall asleep quickly using this method at any time, get up after an hour or two, and go to work with new energy. So, the method can be used by all, the young and the old— billions of people on the earth.

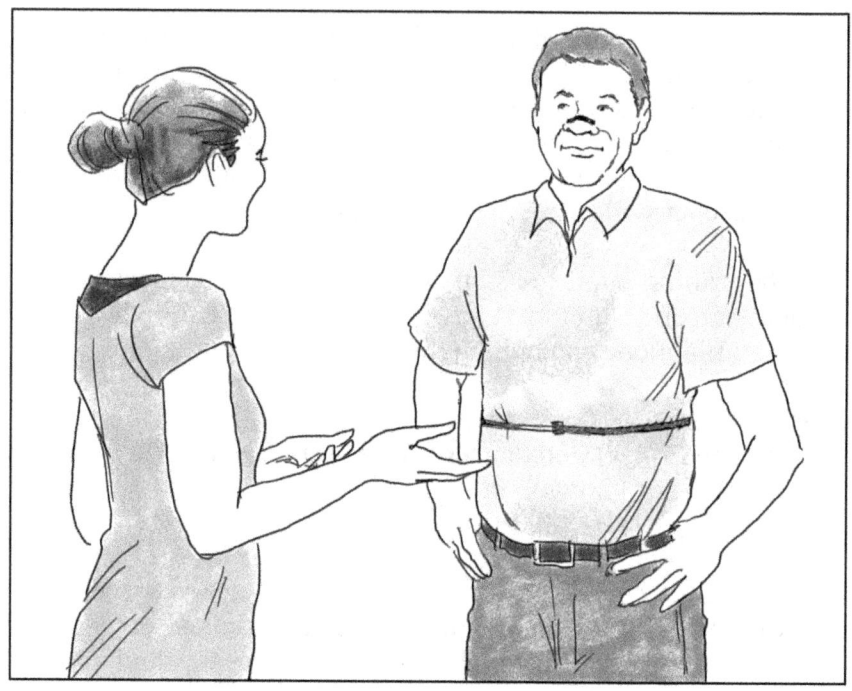

Fig.1.1: Teacher and pupil discuss in the Class

Eve:
I am glad to know that. I will be interested to learn the method. I wish you had been here before Michael Jackson died taking drugs to fall asleep.

Adam:
I am sorry I could not assist Michael Jackson. I did not know about his sleeping problems or his life and death with drugs. I will be happy to teach you the method to enable you learn quickly with a proper use of the devices. The material I am going to cover in the class will be published in a book, so you can review the material at your own convenience, and continue practicing the method on your own until you master the skill. If you have questions or want to practice under my guidance, you are always welcome to get in touch with me. The steps shown in the book as well as in the patent should help you learn the method or master the process on your own.

Eve:
If this is such a useful method to billions of people, why did you not put it into practice years ago?

Adam:
I waited more than seven years to obtain a patent. If I had started teaching the method without a patent protection, the pill or drug makers could have hired someone like you, after you have had the training in the method in one of my classes, and could have set up a parallel organization in a big way, with the money resources they have, and they could have driven me out of business. As you know, that is the name of the game in reality. Then, after I was gone, they could close that part of their business and go back to selling pills or drugs as before and keep making money at the expense of the people's health or life, like the tobacco or gun makers do. Therefore, I had no choice but to wait for the patent all these years.

Eve:
How many years is the patent valid?

Adam:
The patent is valid for twenty years from the date of the original application. Let me explain about the patent and the invention.

Glossary:
*Yoga Nidra*=Deep sleep
*Prasanti loka*=Bliss

# Chapter: 2

## Patent and the Invention

Adam:
Patent (the word originates from the Latin *patere*) means to lay open or make available for public inspection. Patent is a set of exclusive rights granted by a sovereign state to an inventor for a period of time in exchange for the public disclosure of the invention. An invention is a solution to a specific technological problem in the form of a product or process, and it is a form of intellectual property. The procedure for granting patent is placed on the patentee, and the extent of the exclusive rights depends upon national laws and international agreements. A patent application must include one or more claims that define the invention. These claims must meet relevant patentability requirements, such as novelty and non-obviousness. The exclusive right granted to a patentee is the right to prevent others from making, using, selling, or distributing the patented invention without permission.

A patent is not a right to practice or use the invention. It simply provides the right to exclude others from making, using, selling, offering for sale, or importing the patented invention for the term of the patent, which is usually twenty years from the filing date subject to the payment of maintenance fees. A patent is a limited property right the government gives inventors in exchange for their agreement to share details of their inventions with the public. Like any other property right, it may be sold, licensed, mortgaged, assigned or transferred, given away, or simply abandoned. In the United States, only the inventor may apply for a patent, although it may subsequently be assigned to a corporate entity.

The US Constitution authorizes the American patent system in Article One, Sec. 8(8), which states: "The Congress shall have power…

to promote the progress of science and useful arts, by securing for limited times to authors and inventors the exclusive right to their respective writings and discoveries…" And it empowers Congress to make laws to "promote the Progress of Science and useful Arts…"

The laws Congress passed are codified in Title 35 of the United States Code*1 and created the United States Patent and Trademark Office. A patent is requested by filing a written application at the relevant patent office. The person filing the application is referred to as "the applicant." The applicant may be the inventor or its assignee. The application contains a description of how to make and use the invention that must provide sufficient detail for a person skilled in the art (i.e., the relevant area of technology) to make and use the invention. There are requirements for providing specific information such as the usefulness of the invention, the best mode of performing the invention known to the inventor, or the technical problem or problems solved by the invention. Drawings illustrating the invention may also be provided. The application includes one or more claims that defines the scope of protection. Once filed, a patent application is "prosecuted." A patent examiner reviews the patent application to determine if it meets the patentability requirements. If the application does not comply, objections are communicated to the applicant through an office action, to which the applicant may respond. A number of office actions and responses may occur, but eventually a final rejection is sent by the patent office, or the patent application is granted, which, after the payment of additional fees, leads to an issued, enforceable patent.

Thoughts in the mind create signals in the brain and make one act as a result of chemical or biological transformations in the human body. The process to induce instant sleep described here involves particular thoughts in the mind that can create specific signals in the

*1. *See* <u>Prometheus</u> v. Mayo, 581 F.3d 1336 (Fed.Cir) (Under 35 USC 101 Congress intended statutory subject matter to include anything under the sun that is made by man).

brain. An invention as a whole is to benefit a human being, a user of the method, where a series of steps or thoughts are implemented using device(s) to transform*2 particular neurons into a different physical state and function.

In the instant invention "induce instant sleep," thoughts in the mind act as an algorithm in the brain. Thus, the process and the claims described here are directed to cure a natural phenomenon of "intrusive thoughts" streaming into a sick brain, a physical object, and the process repairs particular neurons in the brain by transforming into a different state. In this method, it is self-evident that the process incorporates a fundamental principle (of thoughts or series of acts) in making the brain neurons, the material substance undergo a chemical and biological transformation for a particular beneficial purpose. The process incorporates a fundamental principle and the transformation is central to the purpose of the process, since it transforms brain neurons into a particular or different state by applying the fundamental principle, and it does not preempt the use of the principle to transform any other brain part or transform the same neurons in a manner not covered in this method, or do anything other than transform the specific neurons that can produce melatonin and serotonin. The purpose of the process is to treat human brain neurons. When administering positive signals, the neurons necessarily undergo a transformation. The signals do not pass through the neurons untouched without affecting them. In fact, the transformation that occurs, viz., the effect on the neurons after administering specific thoughts, is the entire purpose of administering the signals:

---

*2. *See* Parker 437 U.S. 584; Funk Bro. Seed Co. 333 U.S. 127; and Mackay Radio & Tel. Co. 306 U.S. 86 (process is patentable under 35 USC § 101. ...when a claim containing a mathematical formula implements or applies that formula in a structure or process which when considered as a whole, is performing a function (transforming or reducing an article to a different state) which the patent laws were designed to protect...A process is not un-patentable simply because it contains a law of nature or algorithm.. if there is to be an invention (even from an abstract idea), it must come from the application of the law to a new and useful end ... while a scientific truth is not a patentable invention, a novel and useful structure or process created with the aid of knowledge of scientific truth may be ... (when the process performs a function)).

the thoughts that are administered provide signals, which become active in the treatment of disease, to a subject. As pointed out, the transformation of brain neurons, a physical substance or matter can be described as occurring according to natural processes and natural law. Transformations operate by natural principles. The transformation here, however, is the result of the administration of thought signals (like a drug) to a subject to transform—i.e. treat—the subject, which is itself not a natural process.

The administering acts are not insignificant extra-solution activity or redundant acts, and the claims are of a transformative method of treatment. The claims cover a particular application of natural processes to treat a disease (or mental disorder). The claims do not preempt*3 natural processes; they utilize them in a series of specific acts.

The inventive nature of the claimed method here stems not from preemption of all use of these natural processes, but from the application of a natural phenomenon in a series of transformative acts comprising a particular method of treatment. A claimed process that transforms a particular substance to a specified different state by applying a fundamental principle would not preempt the use of the principle to transform any other substance, to transform the same substance but in a manner not covered by the claim, or to do anything other than transform the specified substance. It is clear that the method of treatment is patentable subject matter under 35 USC 101.

---

*3. *See* <u>Diamond v. Diehr</u>, 450 U.S. 175, 187 (Their process admittedly employs a well-known mathematical equation, but they do not seek to preempt the use of that equation; rather, they seek only to foreclose from others the use of that equation in conjunction with all of the other steps in their claimed process). See *In re* <u>Bilski</u>, 545 F.3d 943, 954, (Because the claims meet the machine-or-transformation test, they do not preempt a fundamental principle… a definitive test to determine whether a process is tailored narrowly enough to encompass only a particular application of a fundamental principle rather than to pre-empt the principle itself).

Eve:
The law of Congress looks simple and it is clear even to me, a lay person. Why did it take 'all those years' to get patent to your invention?


Adam:
It is a long story. Let me tell you a shorter version and if you want to know more please read the book with the pleadings coming out soon.

# Chapter: 3

## The Patent Examiner

Adam:
In June 2006, I filed the original application for patent in the US Patent and Trademark Office for the process to 'induce instant sleep'. A patent examiner refused to consider or review the method seriously and claimed it was a "mental exercise" and no patent would issue. And, the examiner suggested that I hire a patent lawyer to pursue the patent, if I want. Then, a patent lawyer filed an amendment to my application which is allowed. In May 2007, the patent lawyer and I met the examiner-supervisor and argued that the process effectuates changes in the user's brain neurons, which produces melatonin and serotonin to allow the brain to fall asleep. Although the examiner-supervisor agreed orally that the method could be patentable, he wanted to consult with the "in-house authority" for approval. A few months later, the examiner rejected patent, claiming the method was not patentable under 35 USC 101.

At the end of 2007, I re-filed my application for patent which the rules allow. This time a new examiner, after sitting on it for a year, decided to reject the patent. Then, at the end of 2008, my patent lawyer filed an application called Continuation in Part (CIP) for the patent on my behalf addressing the issues raised by the new examiner. The examiner sat on it nearly a year, and in October 2009 decided to reject it again. Shortly thereafter the patent lawyer and I met the examiner and the examiner-supervisor to discuss the issue. At that time, nearly three and half years after the original filing for the patent, the examiner, for the first time, informed me of a new rule. Apparently, the commissioner for patent had revised the policy in August 2009 to state that 'any change in the brain due to mental thoughts is not patentable.'

Given that the commissioner made a new rule to stop the patent, my patent lawyer lacked trial court experience, and I lacked funds to hire a trial-lawyer, I as a *pro se* filed a case against the commissioner in December 2009 before a federal judge and requested the judge to strike the new rule, which violated my rights.

The US Department of Justice (USDOJ) lawyer filed pleadings on behalf of the commissioner claiming that the new rule did not change the law, nor was a final rejection of patent issued contingent upon this new rule; hence, the trial judge was without jurisdiction or power to decide on the issue of the new rule raised in the case.

In April 2010, the judge did not allow me to present evidence or prove that it was a new rule that violated my rights. And the judge dismissed the case, claiming lack of jurisdiction or power to decide whether or not the new rule had violated my rights. Although the judge has the power under Administrative Procedure Act (APA) to strike the new rule, she sided with USDOJ lawyer and dismissed the case under the pretext the court lacked jurisdiction. The judge knew from my pleadings the method to induce instant sleep is a skill that most people need to acquire (1) for falling to asleep at any time without the use of pills or drugs, (2) beneficial to all people, especially to the professionals or business executives who are on the run and subjected to stress or anxiety, and (3) comes handy for insomniacs or for those who occasionally have trouble falling asleep.

Eve:
I am curious to know what did your application for patent say and why did the examiner reject it?

Adam:
As I said it is a long story. So, let me tell you briefly what transpired between the examiner and me:

Patent examiner inquired me: Are you an expert in this unique 'sleep method' and knew all about body, mind, and spirit.

I informed the examiner: First of all, I am no expert on body, mind, or spirit. I rediscovered a process, an ancient method, which can make anyone go to "*prasanti-loka* or *yoga nidra*"—i.e., fall asleep instantly whenever one wants, day or night, either for a short nap or a long, deep sleep, if one learns to use the process properly. It can work for short naps or for a full night's sleep of eight hours. So, for those who may be interested to learn the method, I can teach them. And before we go into the method that can induce instant sleep, please allow me to give you some background information, both technical and nontechnical, and bring you up to date on the present knowledge of how sleep and health relate.

I am here to discuss with you my application for a patent, which deals with the need for sleep and how to fall asleep without a struggle. And I am here to present to you how one's mental health depends on a good night's sleep, and what one should do to fall asleep whenever one wants, at any time during the day or night, without pills, drugs, or alcohol.

We know that the brain is the control center of the body. It controls thought signals, senses, memory, and the function of cells and organs. The survival of a living being depends on a properly functioning brain. We need it to regulate the functions of the organs—for example, the heart pumps blood, the lungs breathe air, and the digestive system assimilates water and food.

A person's brain requires a sleep cycle including deep sleep (DS) and rapid eye movement (REM) sleep of about eight hours in a twenty-four-hour day-night cycle to function properly. Refer to the study at Harvard Medical School and University of California*4. Also, see a sleep study at Oxford: "Counting Sheep No Aid to Insomnia."*5.

---

*4 …a lack of sleep causes the brain's emotional centers to dramatically overreact... (with) psychiatric disorders... (and) fractures the brain mechanisms that regulate key aspects of mental health... and, sleep appears to restore emotional brain's circuits....

*5 1 in 10 suffers from chronic insomnia and it is estimated that sleeplessness costs the US economy $35-billions a year....

Thus, sleep problems play a key role in a large number of brain disorders. For example, strokes and asthma attacks tend to occur more frequently due to changes in hormones, heart rate, breathing rate, and other changes associated with sleep. Neurons that control sleep interact closely with the immune system, as sleep helps the body conserve strength that the immune system needs. Sleep problems occur in almost all people with mental disorders, including those with depression. A person with depression is often awake during the night and unable to get back to sleep. Extreme sleep deprivation can lead to a seemingly psychotic state of paranoia and hallucinations in an otherwise healthy person and disrupted sleep can trigger episodes of mania or agitation and can result in hyperactivity to a person suffering from manic depression. The National Sleep Foundation (NSF) "Sleep in America" poll found that 74 percent of American adults experience sleep problems few nights a week, 39 percent get less than seven hours of sleep each weeknight, and more than 37 percent (one in three) are so sleepy during the day that it interferes with their daily activities. The sleep problems arise from changes in the brain regions and neurons that control sleep, or from drugs used to control other disorders. Once a sleep problem develops, it can significantly impair a person, leading to confusion, frustration, or depression. Sleep problems are common in many other disorders as well, including Alzheimer's disease, stroke, brain injury, and cancer. Refer to "Lancet Oncology," the international agency for research on cancer, the cancer arm of the World Health Organization*6.

---

*6 Scientists suspect that shift work (night-work) is dangerous because it disrupts the circadian rhythm, the body's biological clock. The hormone melatonin, which can suppress tumor development, normally produced at night. Light shuts down melatonin production, so people working in artificial light at night may have lower melatonin levels, which scientists think can raise their chances of developing cancer. Sleep deprivation may also be a factor. People who work at night are not usually able to completely reverse their day and night cycles. Not getting enough sleep makes immune system vulnerable to attack, and less able to fight off potentially cancerous cells. Certain processes like cell division and DNA repair happen at regular times; but if the body needs to do something done at an unusual time- like producing insulin in the middle of the night to help digest food- that can set off a chain reaction of biological mistakes. The problem is re-setting your body's clock.

Now, let me briefly touch upon the acts in the brain that make one fall asleep or stay awake. Circadian rhythms are regular changes in mental and physical characteristics that occur in the course of a day (*circadian* is Latin for "around a day"). The body's biological "master clock" in the brain controls most of the circadian rhythms. The pattern of waking during the day when it is light outside and sleeping at night when it is dark is a natural part of life's circadian rhythm. Only recently have scientists begun to understand sleep alternating and its relation to daylight and darkness.

A key factor that regulates human sleep is exposure to light or to darkness. Exposed light reaches photoreceptors in the *retina of the eye and creates signals to stimulate* a nerve pathway along the optic nerve from the retina to an area in the brain called the "thalamus-hypothalamus" (Fig. 3.4). There, a special center called the supra-chiasmatic nucleus (SCN) initiates signals to other parts of the brain, including sending excited signals into the cortex (Fig. 3.2), which keeps a person awake. The SCN is the "master clock," a pinhead-sized brain structure that contains about twenty thousand neurons.

This SCN works to set a regulated pattern of sleep cycle. Once exposed to the first light each day, the clock begins performing such functions as raise body temperature, increase heart rate and breathing, and release stimulating hormones like cortisol. The SCN also delays the release of other hormones like melatonin (dopamine), which are associated with sleep onset, until many hours later when darkness returns. The signals from SCN travel to several brain regions, including the *pineal gland,* which responds to light-induced signals by switching off production of the hormone melatonin. The body's level of melatonin normally increases after darkness falls, making a person feel drowsy. The SCN governs functions that are synchronized with the sleep-wake cycle, including body temperature, hormone secretion, urine production, and changes in blood pressure, heart rate, and breathing. Because sunlight or other bright light can reset the SCN, the biological cycles normally

---

Anyone whose light and dark schedule frequently disrupts- including frequent long-haul travelers or insomniacs- could face the same increased cancer risks. The balance between light and dark is very important for your body, and make sure to sleep in a darkened room. Just get a dark night's sleep.

follow the twenty-four-hour cycle of the sun. Disruptions in circadian rhythms increase the risk of heart problems, digestive disturbances, and emotional and mental problems, all of which may relate to the sleep problem.

Melatonin is a natural hormone made by the human body's pineal gland, which is a pea-sized gland located close to the thalamus in the brain. During the day, the pineal gland is inactive. When the sun goes down and darkness occurs, the pineal is turned on by an active SCN to begin producing melatonin and releasing it into the blood. When the SCN works as it should, it results in inviting sleep to the brain. Melatonin levels in the blood stay elevated for about twelve hours, throughout the night and before the light of a new day, when the levels fall back to low during the daytime. Besides adjusting the timing of the body's clock, bright light has another effect: it directly inhibits the release of melatonin.

At this stage, let us look at the drugs that are available to aid sleep. They can shorten the time it takes to fall asleep and reduce awakenings, which increases the total time spent asleep. Possible side effects include feeling tired or drowsy the next day, memory loss, headache, and problems with performance. Sleeping pills can cause strange and potentially dangerous side effects. Those side effects can include dangerous allergic reactions and bizarre behaviors such as sleep eating, walking, and driving—a person will drive a car while not fully awake and then have no memory of doing so.

In a recent research, Dr. Kripke, director of research at Scripps Clinic in US, suggests: "The use of sleeping pills may cause injury to the heart in addition to shortening life and causing cancer."

A new research study conducted at the University of Iceland by a team led by professor Sigurdardottir, published in the journal *Cancer Epidemiology, Biomarkers and Prevention*, shows a link between disturbed sleep and an increased incidence of prostate cancer with severity. The research team reports: "We found that men with sleep disruption were at increased risk of prostate cancer, particularly advanced prostate cancer, when compared with men who did not report any sleep problems."

The study is interesting and important, especially since it found significantly more aggressive cancers in the disturbed sleep group. But we cannot say insomnia causes prostate cancer; whatever is causing the insomnia may be the cause of the cancer. Stress and depression can create disturbed sleep and lower the immune response. Light and disturbed sleep inhibits melatonin production. So it is better to get at a root cause of the disturbed sleep. People try to take melatonin supplements as sleep aids, but the supplements do not replace the amount the brain produces during the night. Research shows that melatonin production at night can help suppress cellular processes involved in cancer growth. The drugs can have varying effects on melatonin production without a long-term solution, nor the ability to disarm the trigger in play with the sleep/cancer link. The only sure thing is to get a good night's sleep. The Harvard Medical School reports that among women participating in the Nurse's Health Study—one of the largest ongoing surveys of health in the world—those who had worked rotating night shifts appeared to have a moderately increased risk of breast cancer.

A careful review of present scientific knowledge in this matter reveals solid proof in support of my method, and it is ahead of its time when compared to the present state of the science as below:

The brain has two hemispheres, and one is dominant.

The two hemispheres communicate with each other one thought at a time.

Any interference from two or more thoughts in the mind at the same time creates havoc within the motor responses of the brain, and the two hemispheres stop communicating—resulting in a split brain that stops processing thought signals. The split brain causes the light switch to "flip off" in the brainstem's reticular activating system (Fig.3.3) and activates the master clock (SCN) to make the brain fall asleep; thus, it helps to cure depression or mental disorders.

Scientists are struggling to implant a protein or gene into the brain from the outside to act as a "light switch" in the brain for treating mental disorders or "fix" depression; and control the sleep/wake state of the brain with a "flip" of the light switch. Science is looking for a solution from outside, but not within the brain. The scientists are unable to locate or "repair" the light switch in the brain that does not work properly. The method I rediscovered presents a solution within the brain and it works if you know how to use the process. This method can "repair" the "light switch" in the brainstem and make it work without an implant or drugs.

"In the Oxford study "Counting Sheep No Aid to Insomnia," the participants tried to fall asleep while counting sheep or looking at a scene, which did not help to induce sleep. If one is counting sheep or looking at a scene, that requires the brain to concentrate on only one element or one thought at a time. The participants in that study did not know how to bring in and connect two or more thoughts at the same time. The "selection of an object, location, or action" to generate positive signals in the mind is important. More than that, it is important to learn, practice, and master the skill as to how to bring two or more thoughts into the mind at the same time. That is the unique process of this method.

Here, I have a few Figures to present to you—see below:

Figure 3.1: A schematic view of the two hemispheres of the brain.

Figure 3.2: A diagrammatic view showing the key parts in the brain where melatonin and serotonin are made.

Figure 3.3: A diagrammatic sectional view of the left hemisphere of the brain looking from the inside; it identifies the locations of excitatory and inhibitory areas in the brainstem. The upper brainstem sends signals into the thalamus to get them excited; then the thalamus sends those excited signals into appropriate regions of the cortex. The lower brainstem cuts off the signals going out of the upper brainstem (when split-brain occurs) and flips the "light switch" off.

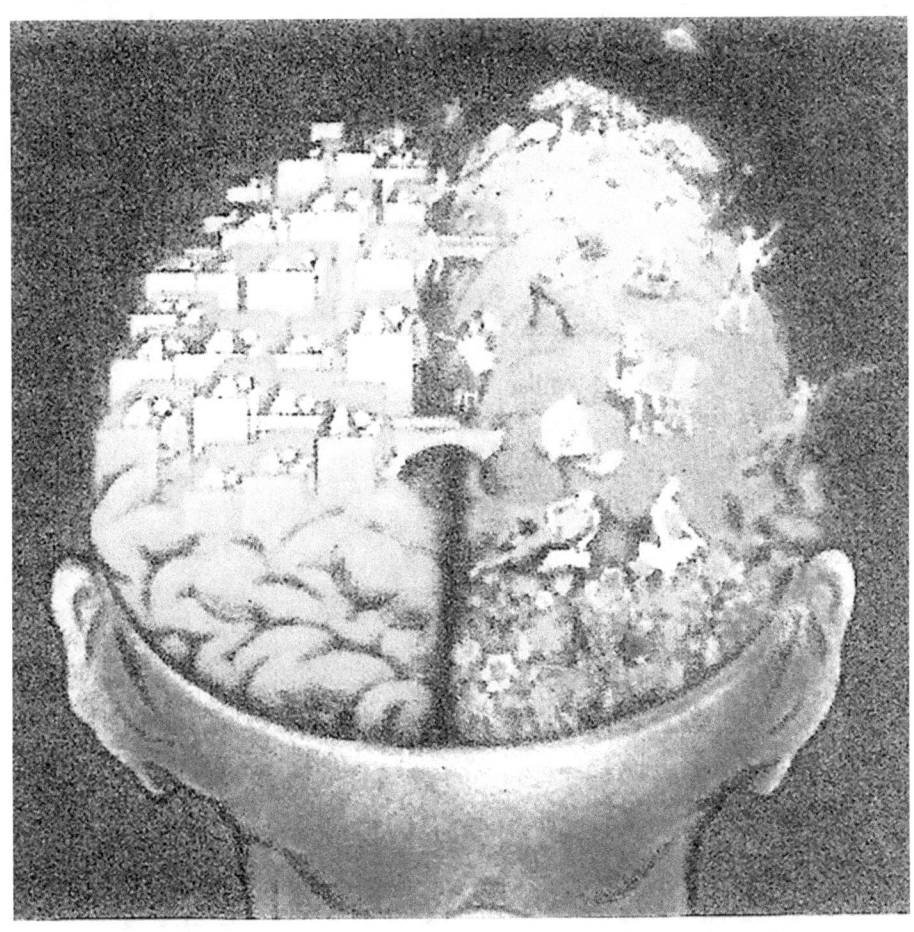

Fig.3.1: Two hemispheres of brain

Guyton & Hall's *Medical Physiology,* 11th ed. Page 719

Publisher Saunders/Elsevier, Philadelphia, Pa.

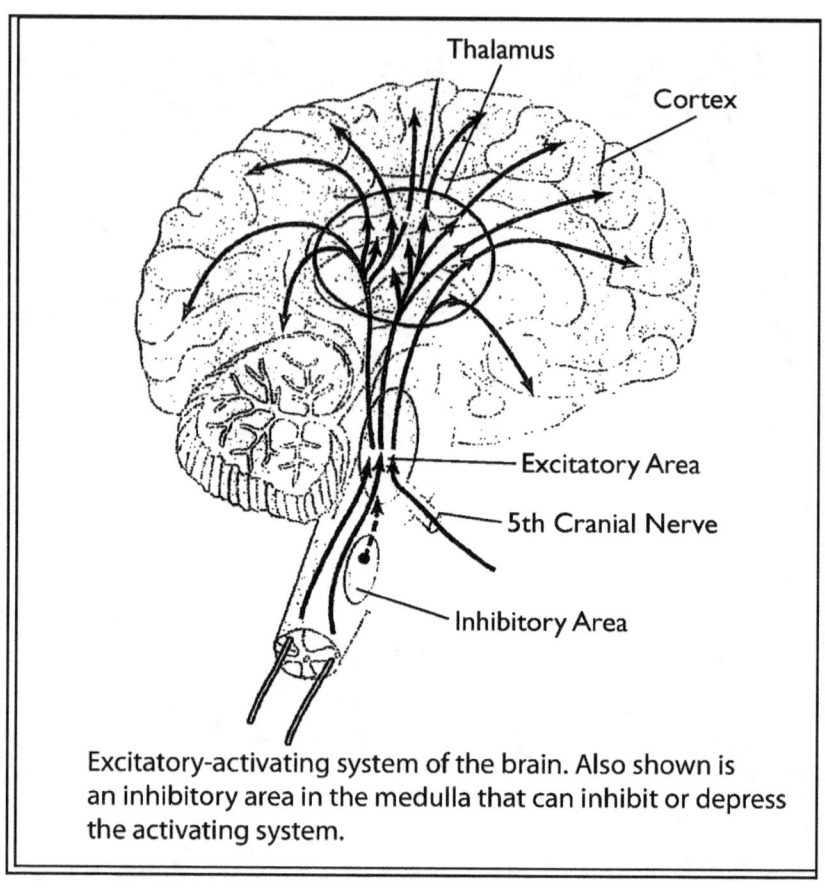

Excitatory-activating system of the brain. Also shown is an inhibitory area in the medulla that can inhibit or depress the activating system.

Fig.3.2: Right hemisphere of the brain as seen from inside.

Guyton & Hall's *Medical Physiology*, 11th ed. Page 729

Publisher Saunders/Elsevier, Philadelphia, Pa.

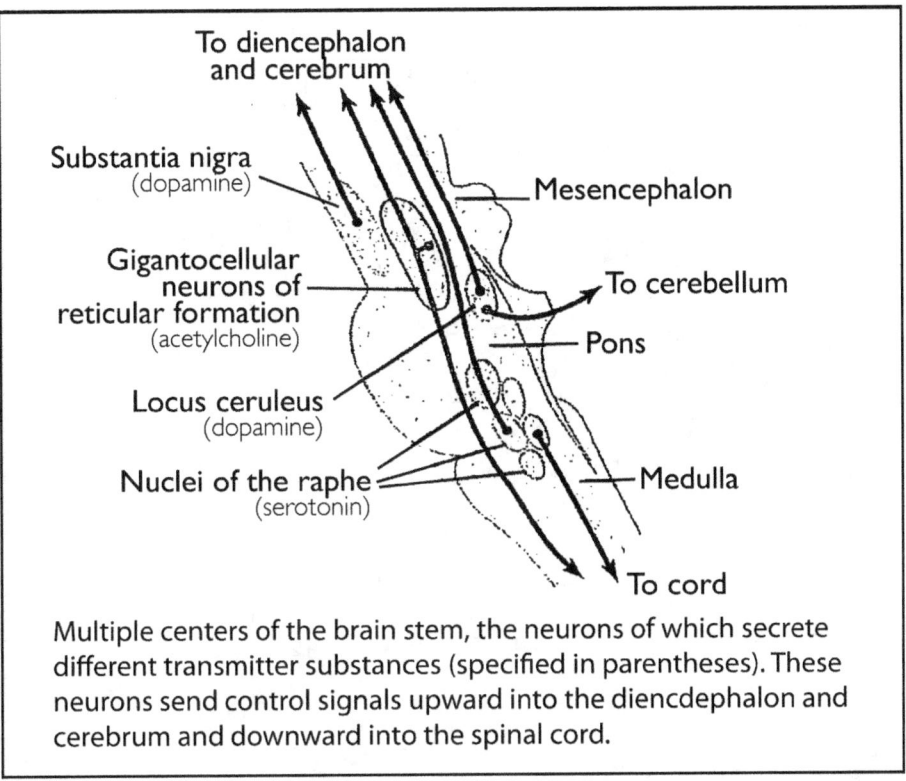

Multiple centers of the brain stem, the neurons of which secrete different transmitter substances (specified in parentheses). These neurons send control signals upward into the diencdephalon and cerebrum and downward into the spinal cord.

Fig.3.3: Left hemisphere of the brain as seen from inside, with the locations for excitatory and inhibitory areas in the brainstem labeled.

Guyton & Hall's *Medical Physiology*, 11th ed. Page 730

Publisher Saunders/Elsevier, Philadelphia, Pa.

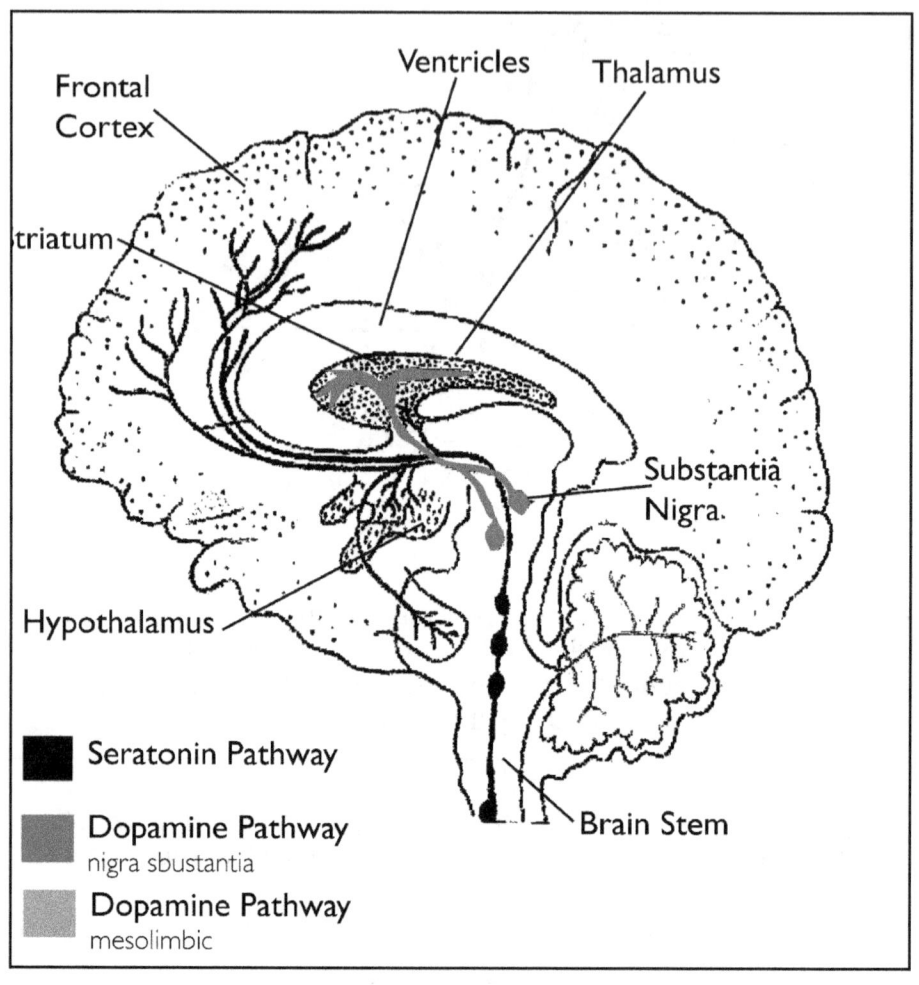

Fig.3.4: Key parts in the brain where melatonin and serotonin are made.

Guyton & Hall's *Medical Physiology*, 11th ed.

Publisher Saunders/Elsevier, Philadelphia, Pa.

Figure 3.4: A diagrammatic sectional view of the right hemisphere of the brain looking from the inside; it identifies the location of the *sustantio nigra,* of which the pineal gland is a part that produces melatonin. The pathways of melatonin into the thalamus are shown where it decreases the signal activity going into the cortex. And it identifies the location of the brainstem, which turns off the light switch when a split-brain state occurs, allowing serotonin to take pathways into the thalamus/hypothalamus and the cortex, and activates the master clock to begin the sleep cycle.

The examiner's next query: When did you discover this method?

I informed him I rediscovered it prior to filing this application for patent in 2006.

Then, the examiner became curious: What do you mean by "rediscovered"?

I explained to him that there is nothing on this Earth that the ancients did not discover millions of years ago. For example, if Jesus is real and you believe he died on the cross and rose to life, it is either a made-up story or he did not die on the cross. As a master *yogi,* he must have used the skill of *yoga nidra* on the cross, and later woke up in the cave. A master *yogi* would not feel pain or spill blood in *yoga nidra* and a *yogi* would find wounds later. So, the method I have rediscovered is like all recent and future discoveries of the man— must be classified as rediscoveries.

Examiner inquires: If so, why did you not help Michael Jackson?

I responded to that this way: First, I did not know he needed help. Second, the Patent Office, i.e. you have stalled the process to issue a patent to the method. If the patent had been issued in a timely manner, I could have publicized the method, and that could have inspired him to contact me.

The examiner sarcastically asks: So, you think it is the patent office with blood on its hands?

I could not deny. I agreed that the patent office certainly should take some responsibility in this case for the suffering of the people including deaths.

Then, the examiner turns around and poses another question to hear my explanation or why I think the patent office is responsible for the delay: How can you blame us, the patent office?

I explained this way: As of now, October 2009, it is more than three years since I made the original application for a patent. The patent office stalled the process, raising all sorts of silly issues, and refused to issue a patent. Under the law "Congress intended statutory subject matter to include anything under the sun that is made by man." That means we know man can make anything under the sun only through principal thoughts in the mind to cause transformation for benefit. You disagreed with that and rejected patent claiming you can find "anything under the sun" as a reason to stop the patent— such as transformation of brain neurons through principal thoughts is not patentable. Then, I went on to explain the process of the method:

This method to induce instant sleep without drugs or pills involves the generation of positive signals in the mind from principal thoughts, which is a mathematical formula; tuning in the new signals to flip off the light switch in the brainstem is an application of that formula. The brain neurons transforming into a different state to perform a function is the method as a whole, which the patent laws must protect. In this method a beneficial result is assured and the benefit is repeatable to a person who learns the skill of the art.

The method involves:

(1) Generating pleasant or positive signal data in the mind using principal thoughts is like writing a song, music, or a computer code on a piece of paper;

(2) Inputting that signal data in the mind into the neuron algorithm of the brain is like inputting data from a computer disc into the processor algorithm of the computer;

(3) Tuning in the signal data in the neuron algorithm of the brain is like processing data in the processor algorithm of the computer; and

(4) Repairing and transforming the neuron algorithm in the brain to function and provide the desired output, a sleep cycle, is like repairing and transforming the processor algorithm in the computer to function and provide a desired output. That's how the Microsoft's processor algorithm came into existence: Microsoft "repaired and transformed" the old IBM processor algorithm of the chips and made the computer work, as in the instant method.

An abstract idea or even a series of mental steps (or thoughts) is patentable if it can create a "novel and useful structure or process" for a useful end. This method is not a game of "abstract functions" or a "mental exercise" for fun. It is a "process" to cure mental disorders with no adverse effects. Thought is not an abstract function; it is the key to everything a human being can do. As we know, a set of thoughts can generate code data to be written for use in a computer; a related set of thoughts can input that data to be processed in the computer; and yet another related set of thoughts can make the output from that data work for the benefit of the man. Similarly, a set of thoughts in this instant method generates data in the mind, inputs that data into a nonworking algorithm in the brain, and keeps processing that data until the algorithm becomes functional and able to produce the desired output: a sleep cycle. The repair and transformation of neurons in the brain to produce this output is not a natural phenomenon, as it can only be achieved using this method.

The examiner asks: How can I verify that the method works?

I responded like this: The physical result or confirmation to the user that something has occurred as a result of this method can be verified by a monitor that records the output signal activity in the brain when awake with streaming intrusive thoughts and when asleep. The output will confirm the result; also, the person will know of the beneficial result upon awakening from a restful sleep. That is true in many other instances, such as in electric shock or radiation treatment, or oxygen therapy, where the person cannot see the input signals or the process of repair and transformation of cells or the output of a different physical state. The final result achieved in the present method is useful, tangible and concrete, and the result is repeatable.

Then, the examiner wants to see evidence: Can you show me research evidence or proof that indeed the neurons transform into a different state during the process?

I answered, yes, I can show evidence. I submitted to you the results from a study conducted on the brains of monks at the University of Wisconsin a few years ago with the help of the Dalai Lama. The MRI images from that study showed improved activity in certain areas of the brain when the monk was in deep meditation, and those areas became inactive when awake.

The examiner wants to know: Do you know if there are any other methods similar to this?

I informed him, none to my knowledge. There is a method and apparatus for auditory and olfactory relaxation using a headset that generates sound and diffuses fragrance; however, it merely provides relaxation, not instant sleep. There is a trophotropic response system, which uses both light and sound to relax; it merely provides relaxation, not instant sleep. And there is an apparatus for projecting "biophilic" natural landscape scenes, or an apparatus for reducing stress that combines music and words. None of those devices make one fall asleep as in this method.

Further, I explained that the method consists of three parts:

(1) *Prasanti-loka* (bliss in mind), the method to induce sleep;

(2) Teaching the method with devices; and

(3) The devices.

Essentially, the method is a process that creates peace of mind and induces sleep. Learning and using the process makes specific neurons transform into a different physical state and enables them to produce melatonin and serotonin without the use of drugs. The devices assist the user in practicing the method and learning the skill of the art to achieve a useful, concrete, and tangible result for benefit.

And I stated the principal concept of the method:

Concentrate upon principal thoughts to calm mind;

Cause split-brain to turn off the light switch in the brainstem which activates master clock (SCN) to make the brain fall asleep.

The first step is to calm the mind of intrusive thoughts and prepare for a sleep cycle—achieve that by calmly visualizing in the mind one principal thought upon the nose device or the breath (or any object, location, action, etc.). That calms the mind. The second step is to split the brain—achieve that by calmly and equally visualizing in the mind, at the same time, two or more principal thoughts upon the nose device, the breath, the diaphragm device, and the movement of the diaphragm (or any object, location, action, etc.). That activates the master clock (SCN) and induces a sleep cycle.

Learning to breathe with the nose device and the diaphragm device on allows one to breathe freely and deeply into the lungs. That could help alleviate mild sleep apnea and the upset stomach—a cause for constipation and peripheral neuropathy which could result in skin problems, urinary problems, and pain in legs (below ankles, toes or elsewhere), and hearing/ vision loss.

It is the principal object of this method to calm the mind and split the brain to induce sleep to a person who otherwise is unable to go to sleep naturally. Thus, the method could help alleviate stress, anxiety, anger, mental distress, depression, mental disorders, or neurodegenerative and neurological disorders, and other health problems such as high blood pressure, hypertension, hot flashes, obesity, and cancer. Any person, irrespective of culture, religion, nationality, sex, wealth, or lack of it, can derive benefit from the method in an inexpensive, dependable, and effective way—not become addicted to drugs.

Then, I showed to the examiner a few more figures that describe the method. The flowchart in Fig.3.5 summarizes the steps involved in the process of the method. The user places a nose band on the nose and places a diaphragm band around the waist. Then, the user lies down and closes the eyes. The user first concentrates on one thought. The user then concentrates on two or more thoughts. As a result, the user then goes to sleep.

The process of concentrating on two or more thoughts with devices creates positive thoughts in the mind, which generate positive signals in the brain; the positive signals, as an input, get processed by the neuron algorithm in the brain to create bliss, and to induce a sleep cycle: both deep sleep (DS) and rapid eye movement sleep (REM). The positive signals focus the attention of the mind away from excitatory negative signals—generated by the natural phenomena of streaming intrusive thoughts into the mind as a result of anxiety, anger, depression, or mental disorders.

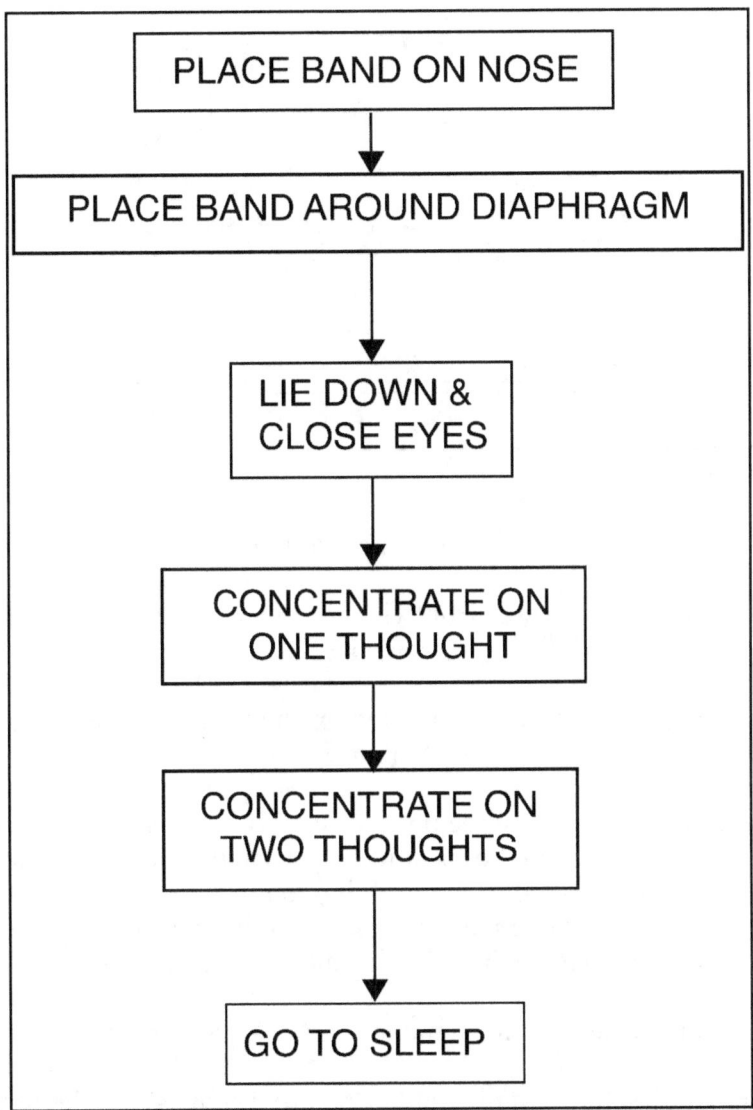

Fig.3.5: A flowchart on the summary of the steps in the method.

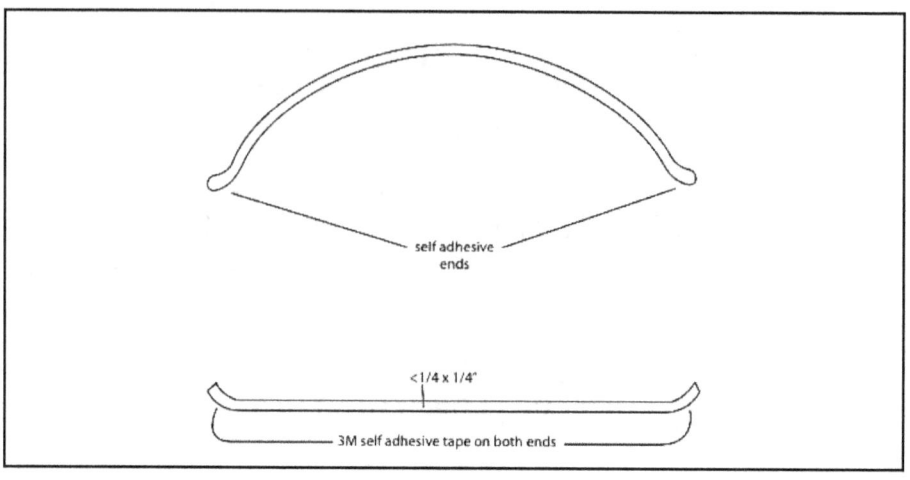

Fig.3.6(**Fig.2***): Above- A front view of the nose-device when put on the nose

Fig.3.7(**Fig.1***): Below- A plan view of the nose-band before put on the nose

Then, further processing of the positive signals in the neuron algorithm will repair and transform the specific neurons in the brain into a different physical state, restoring the brain's ability to produce melatonin, enabling the light switch in the brainstem to flip off, activating the master clock (SCN) in the brain as the output for a sleep cycle.

I informed the examiner in summary, this is what happens:

The method first tunes in pleasant or positive signals into the brain by decreasing the frequency of excited signals in the cortex, and then cuts off the excited negative-signal activity across the neurons in the reticular activating system of the brainstem (Figs.3.2-3.3).

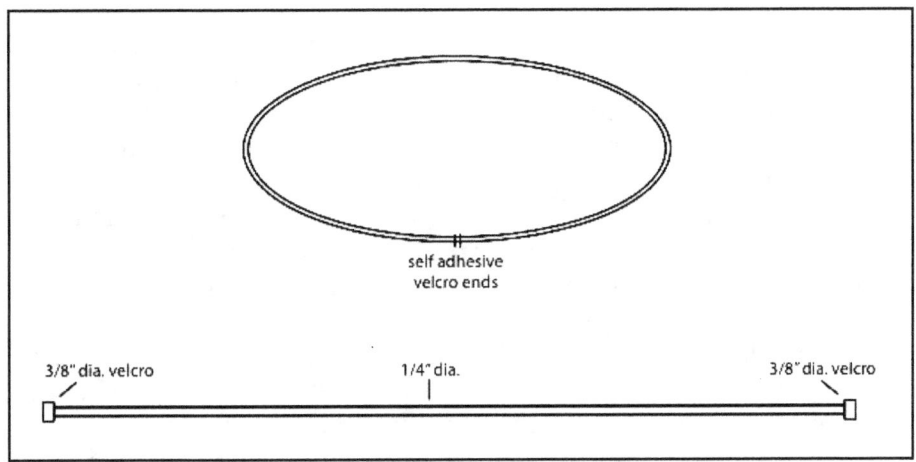

Not to scale, *Patent

Fig.3.8(**Fig.4***): Above- A top view of the diaphragm-device when put on the diaphragm

Fig.3.9(**Fig.3***): Below- A plan view of the diaphragm-device before put on the diaphragm

The initial tuning of the brain is achieved by concentrating the mind upon one principal thought—the device on the nose or inhale/exhale of breath, or the device on the diaphragm or movements of the device on the diaphragm—that helps to calm the mind. The process generates a set of positive signals in the mind, while the information is transferred into the neuron algorithm in the brain to process. This tunes the new signals, replacing the old signals in the cortex, thus decreasing the frequency of excited signals in the cortex and causing a calm state of mind. That process allows the brain to start producing melatonin, a sleep-inviting hormone.

The final tuning of the brain is achieved by concentrating the mind calmly and equally upon two or more principal thoughts at the same time—the device on the nose and inhale/exhale of breath, and/or the device on the diaphragm and the movement of the device on the diaphragm—that helps to cut off all excited signals entering the brain. The process generates two (or more) sets of positive signals in the mind, inputs that data into the neuron algorithm in the brain, and tunes the two sets of new signals to cause an interference that creates havoc in the brain's motor responses, thus splitting the two hemispheres of the brain and stopping them from communicating with each other, causing the "light switch" in the brainstem to flip off and cut all the excited signals coming into the brain. The brain is now able to produce serotonin, which activates the master clock, and puts the brain into a sleep cycle. Thus the brain that was unable to fall asleep before begins to function by utilizing particular neurons in the brain that are repaired and transformed into a different physical state during this process.

The instant method is ahead of its time, as the present knowledge of science is looking to implant a new "light switch" in the brain that will flip on and off to "treat" mental disorders and/or control the sleep-wake state of the brain.

Currently, science is unable to locate or repair the faulty "light switch" in the brainstem that doesn't work. The instant method, however, is able to repair that "light switch" and make it work.

In this method, to induce instant sleep, a person is required to put on the devices, lie in bed (or sit in sofa), and keep the eyes closed to cut off incoming light. The person is required to generate positive signals in the mind while the input data is simultaneously being shifted to the neuron algorithm in the brain. The person must visualize one principal thought about any object, whether it be a thing, location, or action that exists within or outside, such as the device on the nose or breathing air. The person is required to generate positive signals in the mind as the input data into the neuron algorithm in the brain by visualizing two or more principal thoughts about any objects, locations, actions, or combinations that exist within or outside—such as the device on the nose and inhale-exhale of breath or the device on the diaphragm and the movement of the device on the diaphragm or other things that work.

The method to induce sleep will produce a useful, tangible, and concrete result for any person with any sleeping habits. When one learns and masters the method, the positive signals generated in this process will repair and transform neurons in the brain to produce a desired output; it is not a natural phenomenon, as it can only be achieved using this method. The method helps create bliss in the mind and is beneficial to any human being who is unable to become free of intrusive thoughts streaming into the mind due to a brain disorder. The calming positive signals will create a new input into the neuron algorithm in the brain while replacing the excited signals from streaming intrusive thoughts, and the neurons in the brain get repaired or transformed into a different physical state, inducing sleep as the new output. The beneficial result can be confirmed by the change in the recorded output of brain activity when awake and while asleep. The person using the method can sense the benefit or physical result after awakening from restful sleep. The same can be said of the user of sleeping pills except that person gets up tired, drowsy, or with a headache.

The best mode to learn the method is for a person of any variety or heterogeneity of race with vastly different sleeping habits to be willing to learn the art and perform the required steps:

Lie in bed (or sofa) with closed eyes, and practice focusing upon one principal thought, such as on the nose band or any other object, action, etc., until a calm mind is attained with decreased intrusive thoughts in the mind. That practice should continue with different principal thoughts, one at a time, until one thought that works consistently is identified. Then, practice focusing upon two or more principal thoughts calmly and equally at the same time, such as the nose band and the diaphragm band or any one set of thoughts on other objects, actions, etc. until a progressive tuning in of signal interference creates havoc in the brain's motor responses, and splits the brain to make it fall asleep. That practice should continue with the nose band and the diaphragm band or other principal thoughts—two or more at a time—until one set of thoughts that works consistently is identified.

A person who wants to be skilled in the art or who wants to learn the method for benefit should get proper training to acquire the skill.

The method is not a natural process like the natural phenomenon of intrusive thoughts streaming into an insomniac brain due to anxiety, depression, anger, or mental disorder. The method has no environmental and/or learning conditions provided the person is willing to learn. A person willing to learn must identify the nature of intrusive thoughts in order to select appropriate principal thoughts for practice in generating positive signals in the mind. Such a search can help select a set of objects, spots, actions, or combinations to use as principal thoughts in the practice of the method.

I reiterated to the examiner that in this method to induce instant sleep, a person is required to learn to lie in bed (or sofa) and close eyes at the start of the step of concentrating on one thought, and keep them closed through the step of falling asleep to cut off incoming light. The person is required to learn to generate positive signals in the mind as an input into the neuron algorithm in the brain by visualizing one principal thought—concentrate on the nose band or breath or any object, spot, or action that exists within or without. The person is then required to learn to generate positive signals in the mind as an input into the neuron algorithm in the brain by visualizing two or more principal thoughts, such as the nose band and the diaphragm band or any object, spot, action, or combination that exists within or without.

A person who learns the method to induce sleep can produce a useful, tangible, and concrete result whenever the person utilizes the process to decrease intrusive thoughts in the mind, while tuning in the signal interference, which has created havoc in the brain's motor-responses to split the brain. The split brain causes particular neurons in the brain to transform into a different physical state and flip off the "light switch" in the brainstem. The brain then produces serotonin to activate the master clock in the brain and begin a sleep cycle. The result achieved by the instant invention is repeatable for practical application.

Then, I explained to the examiner that the device used in this method comes in two parts. The device to be worn on the nose is shown in Figs.3.6-3.7. It is made of a soft, flexible elastic band configured to fit various nose sizes, with self-adhesive ends to stick to the skin and keep it comfortably on the nose while in use. The nose band is made from rubber or any other suitable material that can elongate or contract sufficiently to facilitate the user breathing freely through the nose and deeply into the lungs. The nose band is reusable a number of times whenever the user wants to utilize the process and fall asleep. The other device to be worn around the diaphragm is shown in Figs.3.8-3.9. In Fig.3.9 the diaphragm band is shown in an open position, with the ends not joined. In Fig.3.8 the diaphragm band is shown in a closed position, with the ends joined, while worn. It is made of a soft, flexible elastic band configured to fit around various diaphragm sizes, with self-adhesive ends to stick and stay comfortably on the diaphragm while in use. The diaphragm band is made from rubber or any other suitable material and elongates or contracts sufficiently to facilitate the user breathing freely through the nose and deeply into the lungs. The diaphragm band is reusable a number of time whenever the user wants to utilize the process and fall asleep.

In the end I gave a summary to the examiner on the method as follows:

(a) Place a nose band on the nose with adhesive ends stuck to the skin.

(b) Place a diaphragm band with the two self-adhesive ends joined.

(c) Lie in a bed (or sofa), turn off the lights, and close the eyes.

(d) Initiate tuning of the brain by concentrating the mind upon one principal thought that generates positive signals in the mind. This replaces old signals in the brain, which will decrease the frequency of excited signals in the cortex, helping to calm the mind and causing the production of melatonin.

(e) Continue tuning the brain by concentrating the mind calmly and equally upon two or more principal thoughts at the same time. This generates a set of positive signals in the mind which causes an interference to create havoc in the brain's motor responses, splits the two hemispheres of the brain, and stops communication between them. That makes the light switch in the brainstem flip off, cutting off excited signals coming into the brain, which helps serotonin production, which in turn activates the master clock, and puts the brain into a sleep cycle.

The examiner wondered if everyone can learn this method.

I answered, yes. We know a person of ordinary skill can learn and acquire a special skill, like bicycle riding, becoming a nurse or brain surgeon, or making a drug, with specific thoughts in mind that create appropriate signals in the human body to act. In the same way, a person of ordinary skill can learn to acquire the special skill of inducing a sleep cycle by generating specific thoughts in the mind which create positive signals in the brain, and that process effectuates chemical or biological transformation of specific neurons to produce melatonin and serotonin required for a sleep cycle.

Eve:
Thank you. I am impressed with your description of the process in response to the quiz of the examiner. The facts and story is clear and makes sense, even to a lay person like me. I am sure the examiner understood your method. If so, what must be the reason for the commissioner to put out a new rule and stop you from getting a patent? Do you think the pleadings you filed in the courts laid out all these facts clearly to make the judges understand your case?

Adam:
Yes, my pleadings are clear and even a 7th grader can understand—you and an expert lawyer can review. The commissioner put out a new rule to stop me from getting a patent protection—please let me explain.

# Chapter: 4

## The Judges

Adam:
As I said before the examiner in October 2009 issued a non-final rejection of patent to my method—'induce instant sleep'—claiming the process is not patentable under 35 USC 101 although the process transforms brain neurons. Thus his rejection contradicts his own finding that satisfies the subject matter requirement to include anything under the sun that is made by man under 35 USC 101. Therefore, to justify his rejection, the examiner simply made up a new rule that a 'transformation of brain neurons due to thoughts' is un-patentable. In support of his position the examiner displays a new rule the commissioner gave him as a guide to follow. And the commissioner would not consider my 'comments' to strike the discriminatory new rule. Therefore, I had no choice, but go to court in November 2009 with a request before the judge to strike the new rule which violated my rights.

In April 2010 the judge dismissed the case with prejudice claiming lack of jurisdiction or power under Administrative Procedural Act (APA). Then, I made a timely appeal to the Court of Appeals for the Federal Circuit and filed the pleadings. I made it clear the trial judge had the jurisdiction or power to strike the new rule because it is a change in the law. And under the law, there is no requirement for a final rejection of a patent to enable the judge to strike a discriminatory new rule. In support, I cited relevant evidence and the law of Congress, US Supreme Court law, and Federal Circuit law. On the basis of willful misrepresentations by the solicitor to the commissioner, in December 2010, Federal Circuit judges denied my appeal and approved the new rule as an "interpretive" rule, although the circuit-judges lacked jurisdiction or power to decide that issue— the issue whether the new rule is 'interpretive or substantive', which the trial judge did not decide when she dismissed the case for lack of jurisdiction or power. The circuit-judges have no-power to decide on an issue that the trial-judge did not decide. That is our Rule of law.

Then, I did not petition the US Supreme Court because that court accepts only about seventy petitions every year out of more than ten thousand. Also, that court never accepts a petition from a *pro se* in a civil case since it is busy protecting the rights of the criminals or "big boys." So the commissioner waited three months to see if a petition would be filed in the Supreme Court, then the examiner entered a final rejection of patent in March 2011 using the new rule, and said:

"Examiner agrees that thoughts produce brain-neuron changes in the brain; however, these transformations are not considered an eligible transformation."

Immediately in March 2011, or within one year from the date of the trial judge's dismissal of my case in April 2010 for lack of jurisdiction, I filed a motion before the same judge to allow the case to proceed to discovery of evidence because the commissioner (and USDOJ lawyer) had committed fraud on the courts using a so called 'interpretive rule' as a 'substantive rule' against me and violated my rights. The judge promptly denied my motion (within a week) and claimed I did not demonstrate clear and convincing evidence of fraud, although the judge was one of the actors in this fraud. Upon appeal, in November 2011, the Federal Circuit judges, apparently being a part of the fraud, agreed with the trial judge that I "failed to show any evidence of fraud" and claimed the trial judge did not abuse power. The court-record makes it clear the trial-judge has the power to decide the case on the merits, but chose not to claiming lack of jurisdiction. This is all a game for the judges and a fraud on the court by a judge is not an abuse of power, either. Thus, between November 2009 and November 2011, a three-year period was lost due to USDOJ and commissioner fraud on the courts. Here I give you a brief account of the fraudulent statements made by USDOJ lawyer and the judge in dismissing the case without allowing me to present evidence:

The USDOJ lawyer said: This court cannot exercise Administrative Procedural Act (APA) jurisdiction to review examiner's non-final rejection...plaintiff attempts to argue that a single sentence in commissioner's interim guidance serves as a substantive rule because it substantively deprives his rights... Even if the examiner is bound by the interim guidance and if plaintiff's patent is finally rejected, he will be entitled to go into a federal court without being hampered by the interim guidance. And the commissioner made it clear it is an interpretive rule, not a substantive rule making...

I asked the judge to review the new rule under APA, and I did not ask the judge to review the non-final rejection. The USDOJ lawyer thinks it is a game and he can twist the facts and law as he pleases knowing the judge would listen and do a favor.

The judge plays the tune in support of the USDOJ lawyer: The way the law is set up, this court has no ability to rewrite the interpretative rule.

Who asked her to rewrite the interpretive rule? I did not. The judge is a master twister, like most of the judges.

The USDOJ lawyer agrees with the twisted version of the judge:

That's correct…The Federal Circuit has the authority to tell the commissioner that the interpretive guidance is wrong.

USDOJ lawyer and the judge knew Federal Circuit will have no power to tell the commissioner the 'interpretive guidance is wrong' when the trial-judge dismisses the case for lack of jurisdiction under APA without deciding the issue whether the new rule is interpretive or substantive.

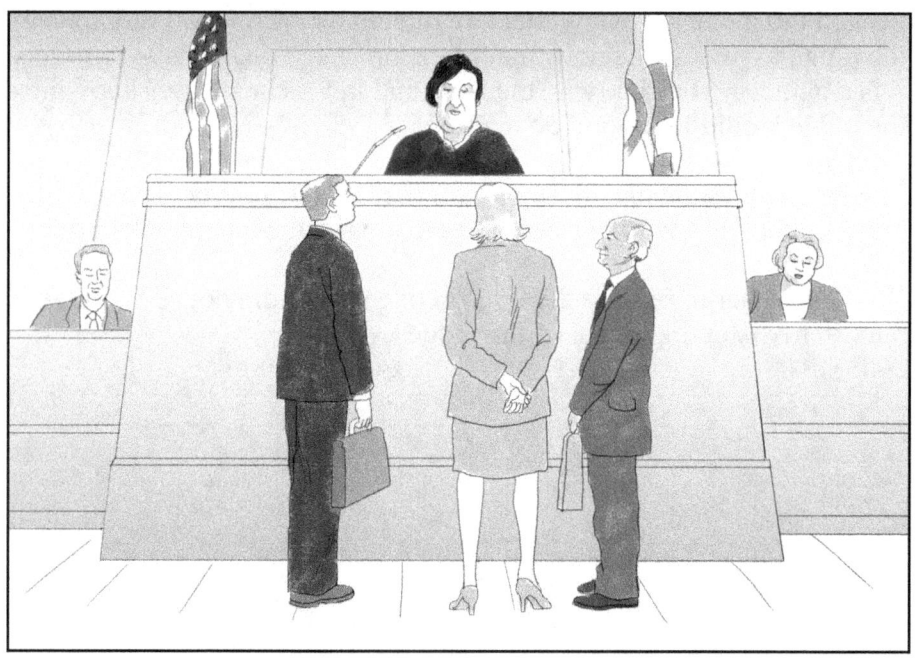

Fig.4.1: Judge in the court with USDOJ lawyers and *pro se*

The judge goes on making irrelevant comments to muddle the record in support of her pre-determined decision: It's not an abstract process where there has been no final rejection [of the patent].

My pleadings made it clear to the judge that a final rejection has no bearing to my case under APA, and my request is to strike an unlawful new rule.

The USDOJ lawyer continues the game: There would be no standing for an individual [applicant] unless there was some reasonable expectation that it [Interim Guidelines] would be applied against them in a detrimental way...

Yes, I made that claim in my complaint with relevant documents attached to show I have the standing because the new rule in the guidelines is being applied against me in a detrimental way. The USDOJ lawyer and the judge knew, but decided to twist the facts and law creating a record in support of announcing their predetermined decision to dismiss my case. The judge did not give me a chance to present evidence or allow me to respond to any of the non-issues the USDOJ lawyer spoke of. The lawyer and the judge knew what they were doing talking in a coded language on non-issues to mask the fraud they decided to commit. I did not ask the court to review a non-final rejection of patent, or my ability to go into a federal court after final rejection of patent is not relevant here. In the present proceedings I asked the court to take jurisdiction in the matter under APA and decide whether or not the new rule or policy is 'substantive or interpretive'—a simple issue. And the court has jurisdiction to hear evidence on that issue and make a rule. Instead, the lawyer and the judge engaged on non-issues making me, a non-lawyer *pro se*, look like a fool and decided whatever they have cooked up behind the scene:

Then, the judge looks at me and says:

The reality of it is that the lawsuit and the motion that you have filed in this court have no legal foundation. As the government has correctly pointed out, you have not yet had a final agency action— the patent has not finally been rejected... without a final action from the agency, you really have no basis to be in this court. The case is dismissed and your motion to set aside the substantive rule is denied. And on April 30, 2010 (see order #**4** below), the judge enters an order: "For the reasons stated in open court, defendant's motion to dismiss is granted and plaintiff's motion to set aside USPTO's substantive rule and enter declaratory order is denied, and it is hereby ordered that this civil action be and is dismissed with prejudice."

"With prejudice" means I am not allowed to re-file the case, again— even when the order is a fraud. In doing so, the judge did not decide whether the commissioner had failed to take a discrete action which is required to be taken upon receiving my "timely filed comments" and repeal the substantive rule or the change in policy that was made effective in August 2009, before notice and public comment under APA @553(c), (d) & (e) and 706(2)*7.

The dismissal of the case for lack of jurisdiction provided a cover to the judge to avoid taking evidence and not decide whether the new rule made effective by the commissioner is substantive or interpretive.

Upon timely appeal to the Court of Federal Circuit, that court decided not to provide me, a *pro se*, with an oral argument knowing the law is in my favor; and the circuit-judges entered a non-precedential order in favor of the commissioner. The non-precedential order means, this decision is only applicable to me, a *pro se*, and the decision can't be cited as the law in any other future cases. Therefore, the fraud on the court committed by USDOJ lawyer, solicitor for the commissioner, and the judges would not see the light of the day and will be buried forever.

---

*7 See Norton, 542 US 55 In Cooper, 536 F.3d 1330 (Fed Cir 2008) (We have also previously held that 35 USC @ 2(b)(2) does not authorize the Commissioner to issue "substantive" rules).

See Merck, 80 F.3d 1543 (A rule is 'substantive' when it 'effects a change in existing law or policy' which 'affect[s] individual rights and obligations').

See Animal, 932 F.2d at 927 (In contrast, a rule which merely clarifies or explains existing law or regulations is 'interpretative').

In Tafas, 559 F.3d 1345 (Fed Cir 2009 en banc) (While the text of the rules sets forth a facially reasonable procedural requirement, we are mindful of the possibility that the Commissioner may in some cases attempt to apply the rules in a way that makes compliance essentially impossible and substantively deprives applicants of their rights. In such cases, judicial review will be available under 5 USC @ 706).

And, in Tafas the Commissioner had to *rescind* the rules that formed the basis of that litigation (both *substantive* and *procedural* new-rules).

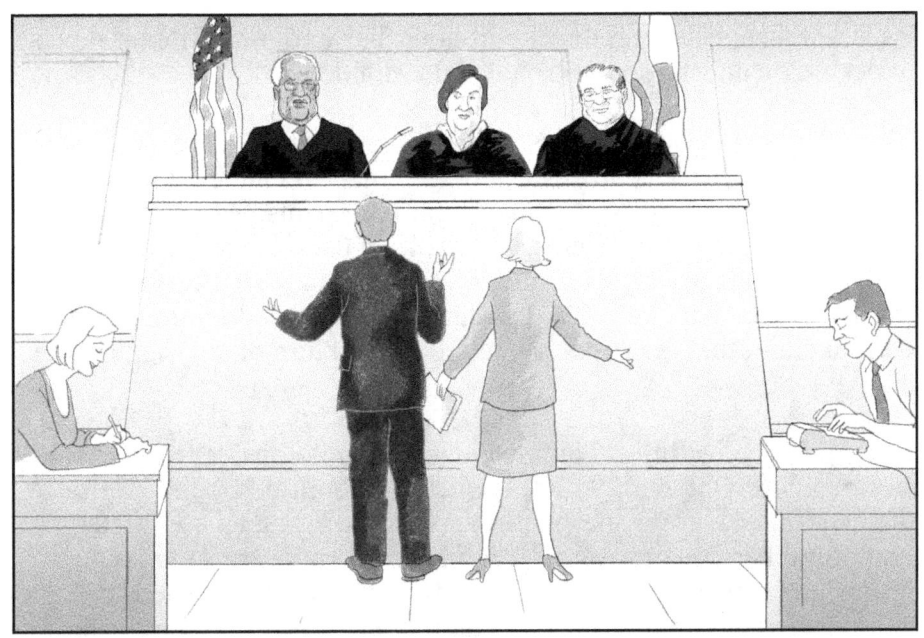

Fig.4.2: Panel of judges with the Commissioner's solicitors

Here, I cite some of the arguments the solicitor for the commissioner made, my responses to those, and the decision of the circuit-judges:

The solicitor for the commissioner: The one sentence, "Purely mental processes in which thoughts or human-based actions are changed are not considered an eligible transformation," in the Interim Examination Instructions for Evaluating Subject Matter Eligibility under 35 USC 101, is not "substantive" rule making, but an "interpretive" rule making under *Animal*, 932 F.2d 920.

I said in my pleadings (see Appendix): The trial-judge did not rule on that issue, whether it is substantive or interpretive, and the judge dismissed the case for lack of jurisdiction. Therefore, solicitor's argument that the one-sentence new rule is "interpretive" is a non-issue in this appeal, and the circuit-court has no jurisdiction or power to decide on an issue the trial-judge did not decide.

The solicitor for the Commissioner: Commissioner has received and considered the comments regarding the [Interim Guidelines of 2009] submitted in response to the request for comments…and the fact that plaintiff had an opportunity to comment on the Interim Guidelines—both before and after the examiner issued an initial rejection of his claims on October 27, 2009—but failed to do so undermines his current claim that the commissioner deprived him of any rights under the APA.

I said in my pleadings: Commissioner did not consider my comments of October 29, 2009, which I submitted by fax before the deadline of November 9, 2009. Again, on August 05, 2010, I submitted comments to the commissioner in response to its notice on Interim *Bilski* Guidance of July 27, 2010. I asked the commissioner to repeal that substantive and discriminatory rule in the Interim Guidance of 2009. The commissioner failed to act on my request and went on to apply the new law against me in a detrimental way…

In my appeal at the Federal Circuit the solicitor for the commissioner made willful false statements that I "failed" to submit comments, therefore, "undermines" my "current claim that the commissioner deprived (me) of any rights under the APA". The documentary 'evidence' of the comments I filed with the commissioner on timely basis is a part of the trial-court and circuit-court record. The judges have simply disregarded the evidence and accepted the false-statements of the commissioner. Then, the circuit-judges enter a non-precedential order to hide/conceal their own fraud on the court and buried it not to see the day light forever:

The circuit-judges said (see order #**3** below): Our decision in *Animal*\***8** is almost directly on point, because commissioner's notice

---

\*8. In <u>Animal</u>, 932 F.2d 920 (Fed Cir) (To establish standing to sue, a party must, at an irreducible minimum, show (1) that he personally has suffered some actual

in *Animal* mirrored the Supreme Court's holding in *Diamond* [so in *Animal* we found] that the commissioner's notice was interpretive rather than substantive. Accordingly, we conclude that the Interim Guidelines [in the present case before us on the 'method for sleep'] are interpretive, rather than substantive, and are thus exempt from… APA… [and] the district court's dismissal was proper.

The circuit-judges <u>admit</u> that the commissioner's notice in *Animal* mirrored the Supreme Court decision in *Diamond* therefore that notice was interpretive. Whereas, in my present case it is a method to 'induce instant sleep' and the commissioner's notice did <u>not</u> mirror a Supreme Court decision to qualify that the notice is interpretive. Therefore, circuit-judges have <u>no</u> basis to "conclude that the Interim Guidelines [in my case] are interpretive, rather than substantive, and are thus exempt from…APA… [and] the (trial)-court's dismissal was proper".

As a matter of law the circuit-judges have <u>no</u> power to decide whether the new rule adopted by the commissioner in my case was interpretive or substantive because the trial-judge did <u>not</u> decide that question when dismissing the case for lack of jurisdiction after refusing to take evidence or allow discovery on the issue. The circuit-judges knew of their willful fraud on the court in entering an unlawful order against me, a non-lawyer *pro se*, which deprived me of liberty or property without due process under the Fifth Amendment. And the judges are aware that their wrongful acts make millions of fellow citizens suffer either for lack of sleep or taking pills to sleep. For that reason, the circuit-judges have decided to enter a non-precedential order to conceal the fraud on the court and keep the decision buried forever with no chance of seeing the day light.

See circuit-judges' order #**3** which said: In *Animal* "the notice, which stated that the PTO 'now considers non-naturally occurring,

---

or threatened injury as a result of the putatively illegal conduct (personal injury), (2) that the injury fairly can be traced to the challenged action (causation), and (3) that the injury is likely to be redressed by a favorable decision (effective relief). In addition to these requirements, standing is further limited to those parties within the 'zone of interests' a particular statute addresses (35 USC @ 101)).

nonhuman multicellular organisms, including animals, to be patentable subject matter within the scope of 35 USC @101,' mirrored the Supreme Court's holding in *Diamond* (447 US at 309)... [so] this court...find[s] that the USPTO notice was interpretive rather than substantive." Whereas, in the subject matter of my case there is (1) no ruling from the Supreme Court to mirror that "Purely mental processes in which thoughts or human-based actions are changed are not considered an eligible transformation", and (2) nor a finding of the trial-judge whether that new rule is interpretive or substantive based on the evidence. For that reason, the circuit-judges' order #**3** which concludes "the Interim Guidelines are interpretive" amounts to a fraud on the court and/or a void order entered without power.

Then, on March 23, 2011, the examiner enters "a final rejection of patent" using the circuit judges' void order #**3** and the new rule that 'purely mental processes in which thoughts or human-based actions are changed is not considered patentable' while accepting 'thoughts produce change in the brain'.

On March 28, 2011, I filed a motion before the trial-judge to allow the case to proceed under APA as a result of the fraud on the courts by the commissioner, who misrepresented a substantive new rule as an interpretive rule, received approval of the court, and turned around to use that so-called interpretive rule as a substantive rule against me in a way to make compliance essentially impossible and substantively deprived my rights. So, judicial review is available under 5 USC @ 706". See Tafas, 559 F.3d 1345 (Fed Cir 2009 en banc)*7.

The trial-judge, on April 7, 2011, denied my motion for relief converting the fraud on the courts as 'commissioner's legal position which is accepted by the courts'. So, the fraud on the court if accepted by a judge becomes a legal position—that is the equal justice.

As a matter of fact, the fraud is not based on the legal positions of the commissioner. The fraud is based on (1) the misrepresentation to the courts that the new rule is interpretive, then turn around to use it as a substantive rule in depriving my rights, and (2) the false statements made to the courts that "the fact that plaintiff (the *pro se*) had an opportunity to comment on the Interim Guidelines—both before and after the examiner issued an initial rejection of his claims on October 27, 2009—but failed to do so…"

I pointed out to the circuit-judges that the trial-judge had converted commissioner's fraud on the courts into a legal position, and the judge made a new law from the bench in a *pro se* case thrashing the law of the Congress, and made the APA a dead letter.

The solicitor for the commissioner: The trial-judge did not abuse power to deny relief in this case.

The circuit-judges on November 10, 2011 (see non-precedential order #**1**): The trial-court did not abuse its discretion in determining that the plaintiff "failed to show evidence of fraud", and thus "we affirm".

The evidence is in the court record. What-else can I, a *pro se*, do to show evidence when the judges are acting blind and refuse to allow me to present evidence. The judges knew that "fraud consists of anything calculated to deceive…by a single act…suppression of truth or suggestion of what is false…" And the judges know that "those who act without jurisdiction face liability for damages" under US Supreme Court ruling in *Stump*, 435 US 349, and under other laws. Here, if what the USDOJ lawyer and the solicitor for the commissioner did is not the misrepresentation or fraud on the court— what is it, a noble act?

Under the guise of an interpretive rulemaking, commissioner has effectively put out a substantive rule that "purely mental processes in which thoughts or human based actions are changed are not considered an eligible transformation" to stop me from getting a patent; and *no* court in the land has *ever* said that. The commissioner's in-house authority simply made this up…as if they can take any position under the sun, with the blind support of the judges who act like gods and look down on the people—that is the status of 'We, The People'.

Eve:
So you were involved in a long fight for the patent—how many years?

Adam:
It was a seven and a half year fight, and the examiner could have dragged on that fight for another twelve and a half years and said good-bye if given a chance. There is no one to question or control the acts of these government agents—a kind of Mafia.

Eve:
It appears the judges clearly look the other way in a non-lawyer *pro se* matter and lend support to the government agents who may have committed the wrongful acts—am I correct?

Adam:
Yes. The judges are government agents—for life. They act like gods, giving themselves complete immunity for all acts, whether wrongful or criminal—as long as they are not caught. The judges always protect one another like a Mafia. And the judges protect other government agents giving them immunity for official acts—even when an agent destroys, falsifies or twists the evidence or the law to cover up wrongful acts. In fact, judges freely twist the laws at will—the laws enacted by Congress—or make new laws from the bench to justify their wrongful acts. In my case, when I went to the court for relief from the wrongful acts of the patent examiner, the judges committed fraud on the court in support of the patent examiner by twisting and disregarding the law of Congress. Such corrupt acts made me lose half of the 'seven and a half years' lost in securing the patent.

Eve:
I did not understand why the judges enter non-precedential orders.

Adam:
That is an order which applies only to me, a non-lawyer *pro se*, and to no one else in the future. That meant to get rid of my case while letting millions of Americans suffer sleeplessly or taking the pills.

Eve:
That sounds like the ruling made by the five judges in *Bush v. Gore* in 2000, which stopped the vote count in Florida and let Bush become the president—am I correct?

Adam:
Yes, that ruling was non-precedential too. You know, that stupid and irresponsible decision hurt millions of people and wasted trillions of dollars on an unnecessary war in Iraq. And none of those responsible for inflicting that injury were ever investigated or prosecuted.

Eve:
What is the crime for which any of them could be prosecuted?

Adam:
Congress should have, and still can, investigate whether or not those five judges had the power to stop the vote count in Florida, thus violating the rights of millions of citizens in Florida and in America. Then, they could find out how these judges could usurp the power and enter a non-precedential ruling, knowing that ruling violates the rights of millions of Americans. And Congress could have investigated why and how Bush got us into the Iraq war, which ruined our economy.

Eve:
Where is the crime?

Adam:
A thorough investigation is the first step, and the evidence could lead to a possible crime.

Eve:
Do you think the judges have violated your own rights as well as the rights of millions of Americans in doing what they did in your case? If so, do you think Congress should investigate the wrongful acts of the US agents— the commissioner for patent, the lawyers, and the judges?

Adam:
Yes; no one is above the law. If no one cares to investigate the acts of the corrupt judges, the criminals will prevail, like the drug-gangs in central-America or Afghanistan or here.

Eve:
So, how did you get the patent in the end?

Adam:
A nonprofit organization called PIIPA helped me find a new patent lawyer who is smart and practical, and he prosecuted for the patent without a fee. The commissioner knew of the wrongful acts of the USDOJ lawyer, his solicitor and examiner, and of the judges; and he knew of possible hearing by the Congress in the matter. So, all these factors made the commissioner to allow his examiner do the right thing. In the process, the examiner delayed another year before acting in December 2012. Thus, a total of seven and a half years were lost due to the wrongful acts of the patent office while millions suffered.

Eve:
I bet it would be interesting to review the court record related to this case and find all the details on the acts of the USDOJ lawyer and the judges.

Adam:
Yes, I think so, too. That is the reason I prepared a small book with illustrations that tells the story—what the agents or servants of the people do to the little people, the individuals. To learn more of the story, you can review the court record later. As a matter of fact, the solicitor for the commissioner who is involved in the fraud on the courts is appointed as a federal circuit-judge.

Eve:
Does that tell you "fraud pays"?

Adam:
Yes, in the short run of the drama it pays; in the long run it is hard to see how the fraud can prevail.

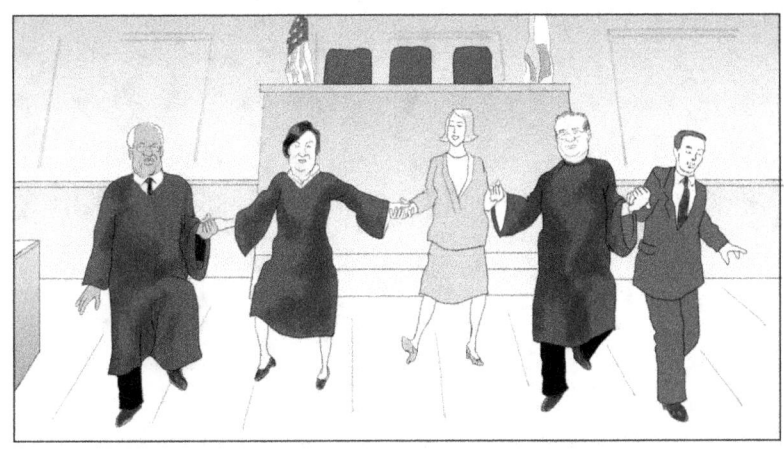

Fig.4.3: Judges and Attorneys sing and dance

Be aware, we are the supreme in the land of free
Be aware, we are the constitution
Be aware, we are here for life
Be aware, we are the gods
Be aware, we are with immunity
Be aware, we are drunk with power
Be aware, we are blind to truth/justice
Be aware, we are free to twist or create law
Be aware, we are free to make law of Congress a dead letter
Be aware, we are free to make the president
Be aware, we are free to do wrongs or fraud on the court
Be aware, we are free to make day into a night or night into a day
Be aware, we are free to protect criminals and big-Boys
Be aware, we are free to see corporations as people
Be aware, we are free to see people as nothing
Be aware, we are free to listen to corporations, not to people
Be aware, we are free and never listen to a pro se!

# Chapter: 5

## Method to Induce Instant Sleep

Adam:
Now, let us get back with the learning part of the process.
Adam begins to teach addressing the class:
I welcome to you all. I am glad to see you here willing to learn.
Please sit relaxed and comfortable.

Before you get settled, take off your jacket and put it on the sofa or bed. And, please come to the front one by one and take a package I have for you—I will tell you what to do with it in few minutes. After few minutes—I hope everyone got a package. Now, let us open the package and see what we got. I find two small bags—please, all of you do the same as I do and find out what is in the package.

Now, let us open the small little-bag and see what is in it—I find one small rubber band and two strips of tape. I hope you find the same. Let me explain what to do with these three pieces. The rubber piece is the nose-band and that goes on your nose—not in the nose. The strips of tape go on the two ends of the nose-band. This is how we should do it: peal the cover off of the tape on its 1st face and stick the tape on to the flat surface of the nose-band at one end; repeat the same process at the other end—make sure it goes on the same side of the flat surface of the nose-band like at the other end. That makes one nose-band with tapes on both ends. Now, peal the cover off of the tapes on the faces you can touch or see; then, holding the ends of the nose-band in your hand-fingers let it arch over your nose, near tip of the nose, and while stretching the band press it on to your skin at both ends and stick it—at the bottom of the nose-bone or arch, securely. Please watch me do it, or raise your hand I can come and show you.

Next, let us open the small second bag and see what is in it—I find one long rubber band, two Velcro buttons, and two strips of tape. I hope you find the same. Let me explain what do to with these pieces. The rubber piece is the diaphragm-band and that goes on your diaphragm, above the waistline, similar to a belt for your pants—but this has no holes or a buckle. The Velcro buttons, male and female, or the two-pieces of tapes are to be used to tie the diaphragm-band ends—like you tie belt with holes and buckle. First, you size the diaphragm-band to fit comfortably over your diaphragm (with your shirt on)—not too tight or loose. Then, peal the covers off of at the back of Velcro buttons and stick one on each end of the rubber band. Now, it is ready for use—put it on the diaphragm joining the male-female ends of the Velcro button. Alternately, if you are not prepared to cut the rubber-band (with a scissor) to size and make it an exact fit, you can stick the tapes at both ends—one piece on the inner face of the rubber-band at one end and the other piece on the outer face of the rubber-band at the other end. That way when you join the diaphragm-band together to make a good fit you can overlap the band and let the tape stick to hold the band in place. Please watch me do it, or raise your hand I can come and show you. I will give you few minutes to get this done and we will start practicing the method.

After few minutes—I hope every one of you is ready with a nose-band on the nose, and a diaphragm-band on the diaphragm. Please watch me: I have put on a nose band and a diaphragm band—raise your hand if you have a question. I do not see any hands up. I hope you did it all right so far.

Now, I request two volunteers, a man and a woman—please come to the front and be seated on a sofa and on a bed closer to me, facing the class. After few minutes—please tell me your names and sit down in the sofa or on the bed, whichever you prefer. I will teach the steps involved in the process and show you how to practice the method properly. I will repeat these steps. The rest of you please watch them do it, or do it yourself while listening to me—see if the steps work for you.

Are you ready to go to sleep? Remember, first the lights should be turned off to make the room dark, like at night. Here, in this class I am going to leave a dimmer light 'on' near me, so you can see me and these two, if required. Before I turn off the lights, you should sit down in a sofa or lie down in a bed, relax, be comfortable closing your eyes, and listen to my instructions. I will give you a couple of minutes before I turn the lights off. After few minutes—now the lights are off, so let us do this: Calmly visualize or see in your mind the nose band…inspect and see how it is sticking to the nose…go ahead and see the nose band in your mind.

Calmly sense or see in your mind the breath through your nose, the flow of air in and out through the nostrils…go ahead and see the breathing in your mind.

Calmly let your mind travel down and visualize or see in your mind the diaphragm band, especially the point where the two ends of the band are joined…go ahead and see the diaphragm band in your mind and take a minute to inspect the joint of the ends.

Calmly visualize or see in your mind the rhythm or movement of the diaphragm band at the joint as you breathe…go ahead and see the movement or rhythm in your mind.

Please repeat that process within your mind, going from the nose band to the diaphragm band as many times as you want, and figure out which one or two things you like the best out of the four things. Now, I will keep quiet to give you time to repeat the process on your own a few times and see if you can fall asleep doing only this first step. If it works, that is great and you may not require learning the second step in the process.

For those of you who did not fall asleep during the first step, I will show you the second step in the process after a few minutes. That should make you fall asleep, provided you do it properly. I am sure this one lesson will not make you an expert in this method. You may have to keep doing it until you master the skill and are able to induce instant sleep.

Now we should try the second step. I do not know how many of you fell asleep. I am sure a number of you are still awake and wanting to learn the second step in the process. So let us get started.

I hope those of you still awake are able to identify which two things out of the four you feel comfortable with. What I mean is, at this time we know of four items you can visualize in your mind: nose band, breathing, diaphragm band, and movement of diaphragm band (near the joint).

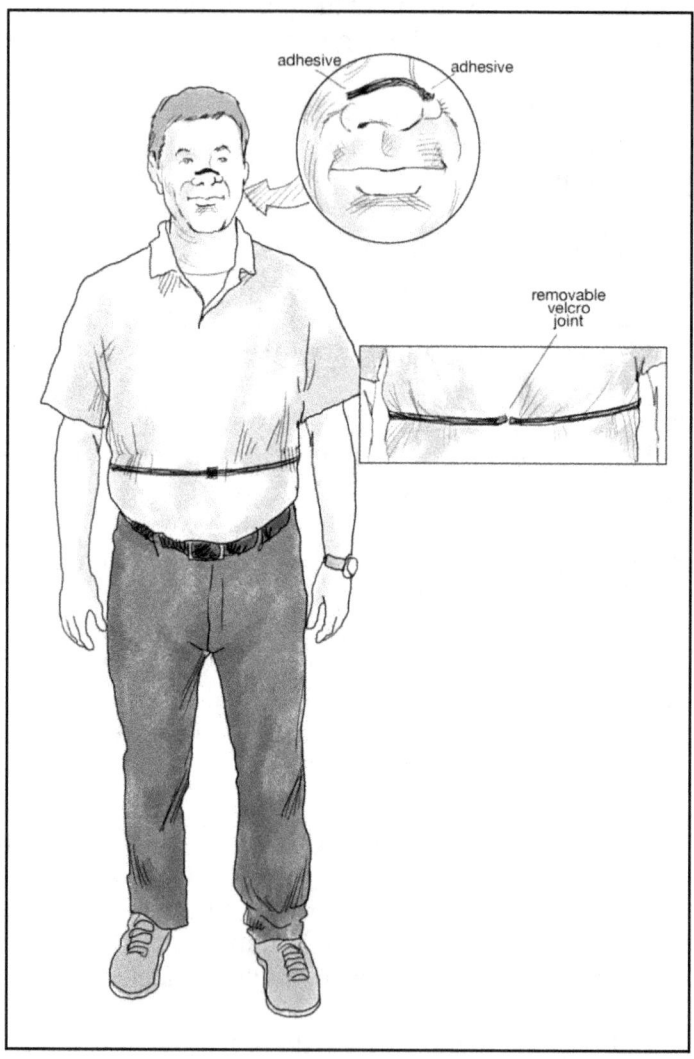

Fig.5.1: Nose band and Diaphragm band in place

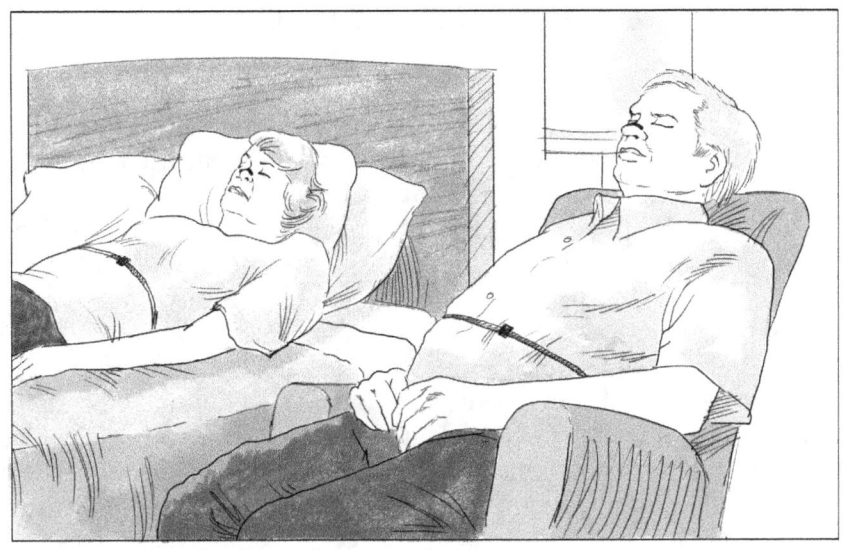

Fig.5.2: Woman and Man practicing the Method with Nose and
Diaphragm bands in position

So pick any two of these four to use in the second step of the
process. And let me say this: if you feel comfortable enough to
visualize in your mind the nose band and the diaphragm band, try
these two in the second step; or if you are comfortable using the
nose band and breathing, that's fine, too. Or, if you want to, you
can pick the diaphragm band and the movement of the band—
that's fine.

So, assuming you have made your pick, I will proceed in this manner:

Calmly begin to visualize or see the nose band in your mind; keep
doing that until you feel ease, as if it is part of your nature.

Calmly begin to visualize or see the diaphragm band in your mind
while continuing to see the nose band in your mind at the same
time—understand, it is not easy to do that. But keep trying until you

acquire that skill and are able to see both bands in your mind at the same instant.

The moment you hit that, seeing it precisely in your mind, you fall asleep at that instant. You will not know what hit you until you get up the next morning. That's the second step. By the way, you can keep the nose band and diaphragm band on you while sleeping and can remove them next morning for reuse, later. In fact, you may not require these bands once you have mastered the skill.

Now I will leave you on your own to continue trying this step again and again until it works for you. If it does, that's fine; otherwise, join me in the next class and continue to practice. You can also register for an Internet class near you and continue the learning process until you master the skill.

I will be happy to continue discussing your questions.

\*\*\*\*\*\*\*\*\*\*

A few days later telephone rings. Adam answers the phone- Hello!

Eve:
I want to thank you teacher Adam for the lesson. I read your book and understood it sufficiently enough to be able to practice the skill on my own with the devices every night; and sometimes I do it during the day whenever I find time to rest and do my professional work refreshed. I am thrilled to report—the method works for me and I am sleeping eight hours a night, and no more pills. And I hope to master the skill in the next few weeks or even sooner by keep practicing until the process becomes a part of me as second nature, like my singing and dancing. In the beginning I had to struggle a bit at every step on the way, especially with the two or more thoughts into my mind at the same instant and cause the split-brain to stop the two-hemispheres from talking to one another. I think that step seem to be difficult to learn and master it quickly. I must say I am very close to the goal post.

Adam:
I am so pleased to learn the good news. I have been looking forward
to hearing from you, and I am glad to hear from you. Do you know if
any of your fellow artists or other friends who might have a problem to
sleep?

Eve:
Yes, I do.

Adam:
If you have the time and wish to help some or all, please let me know.
I will assist you how to be a teacher for them.

Eve:
Yes, I can find time to help my fellow artists— there are many that
can use this skill for their benefit.

Adam:
So, you be the teacher for the artists—being on the cover of the Book
in the next edition.

Eve:
OK, I am in.

# Appendix

US008323175B2

(12) **United States Patent**
Mikkilineni

(10) **Patent No.:** **US 8,323,175 B2**
(45) **Date of Patent:** **Dec. 4, 2012**

(54) **METHOD AND APPARATUS FOR INDUCING SLEEP**

(76) Inventor: **Maheswar R. Mikkilineni**, Washington, DC (US)

( * ) Notice: Subject to any disclaimer, the term of this patent is extended or adjusted under 35 U.S.C. 154(b) by 0 days.

(21) Appl. No.: **13/188,420**

(22) Filed: **Jul. 21, 2011**

(65) **Prior Publication Data**

US 2011/0282131 A1 Nov. 17, 2011

**Related U.S. Application Data**

(63) Continuation of application No. 12/259,285, filed on Oct. 27, 2008, now abandoned, which is a continuation-in-part of application No. 11/999,349, filed on Dec. 5, 2007, now abandoned, which is a continuation-in-part of application No. 11/449,519, filed on Jun. 8, 2006, now abandoned.

(51) **Int. Cl.**
*A61M 21/00* (2006.01)

(52) **U.S. Cl.** ...................................................... **600/26**
(58) **Field of Classification Search** ............. 600/26–28; 128/897, 898
See application file for complete search history.

(56) **References Cited**

U.S. PATENT DOCUMENTS

7,422,014 B1 * 9/2008 Smith ...................... 128/204.23
2008/0319277 A1 * 12/2008 Bradley ...................... 600/301
* cited by examiner

*Primary Examiner* — Samuel Gilbert
(74) *Attorney, Agent, or Firm* — Kenneth H. Ohriner; Perkins Coie LLP

(57) **ABSTRACT**

Method to induce sleep, using devices that are worn on the nose and around the diaphragm. The nose-band is made of a soft, flexible and elastic material, such as perforated rubber, and is configured to fit onto the nose of a user. The diaphragm-band is made of a soft, flexible and elastic material, and is configured to fit over the diaphragm of a user.

**7 Claims, 4 Drawing Sheets**

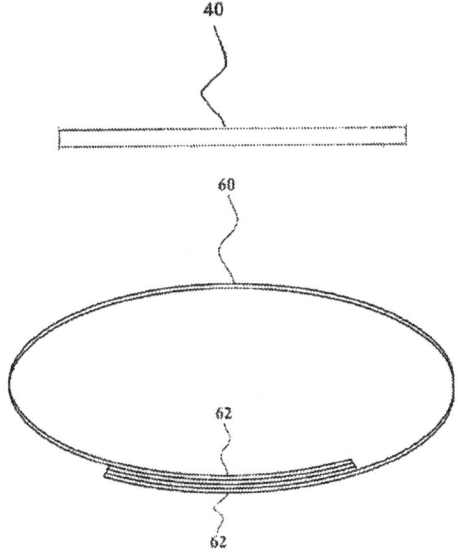

40

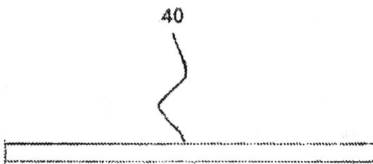

## Fig. 1

40

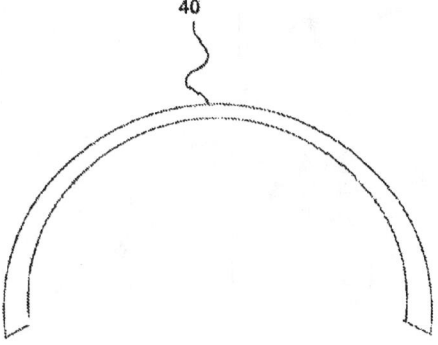

Fig. 2

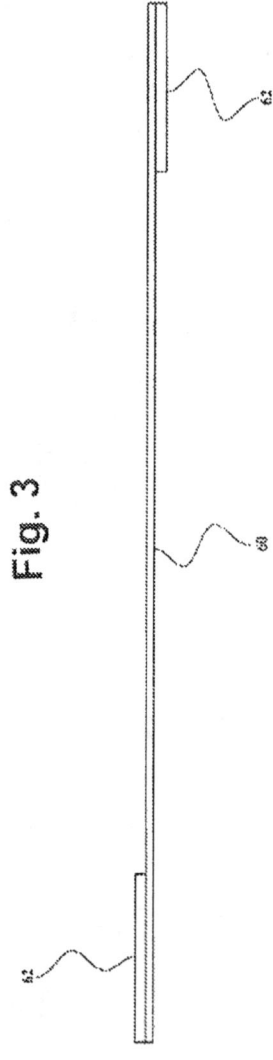

Fig. 3

64

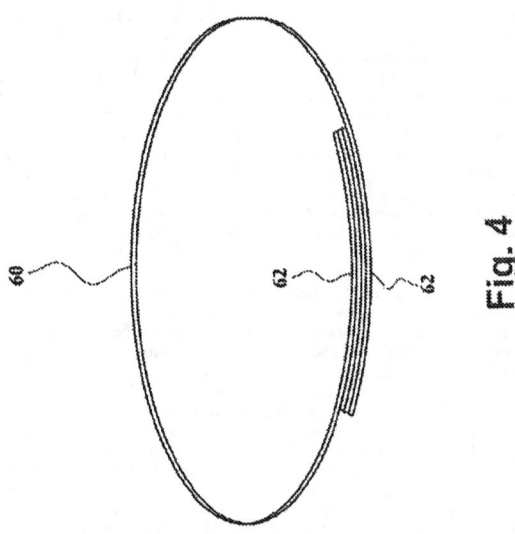

Fig. 4

# METHOD AND APPARATUS FOR INDUCING SLEEP

## PRIORITY CLAIM

This application is a Continuation of U.S. patent application Ser. No. 12/259,285 filed Oct. 27, 2008 and, which is a Continuation-In-Part of application Ser. No. 11/999,349, filed Dec. 5, 2007, and now abandoned, which is a Continuation-In-Part of application Ser. No. 11/449,519, filed Jun. 8, 2006, and now abandoned. These Applications are incorporated herein by reference.

## BACKGROUND OF THE INVENTION

The present invention relates to methods for inducing sleep, without the use of drugs.

Sleep-problems play a key-role in a large number of brain disorders. For example, strokes and asthma attacks tend to occur more frequently due to changes in hormones, heart rate, breathing rate, and other changes associated with sleep. Neurons that control sleep interact closely with the immune system—sleep may help body conserve energy that the immune system needs to mount an attack. Sleep problems occur in almost all people with mental disorders, including those with depression and schizophrenia. A person with depression is often awake in the night and unable to get back to sleep. Extreme sleep deprivation can lead to a seemingly psychotic state of paranoia and hallucinations in an otherwise healthy person, and disrupted sleep can trigger episodes of mania-agitation and hyperactivity, to a person with manic depression.

The National Sleep Foundation's (NSF) sleep in America poll found that 74% of American adults experience sleep problems a few nights a week or more, 39% get less than seven hours of sleep each weeknight, and more than one in three (37%) are so sleepy during the day that it interferes with daily activities. An article 'Counting sheep no aid to insomnia' published in January 2002, on the findings of Oxford study on sleep, reported that "1 in 10 suffer from chronic insomnia and it is estimated that sleeplessness costs the US economy $35 billions a year . . . ." The brain requires a sleep-cycle, deep sleep (DS) and rapid eye movement (REM) sleep, of about eight hours in a 24-hour day to function properly. A recent study at Harvard Medical School and University of California concludes" . . . a lack of sleep causes the brain's emotional centers to dramatically overreact . . . (with) psychiatric disorders . . . (and) fractures the brain mechanisms that regulate key aspects of mental health . . . and, sleep appears to restore emotional brain's circuits."

Currently, there are several prescription drugs available to aid sleep. They can shorten the time it takes to fall asleep and reduce awakenings, which adds to total time spent asleep. Possible side effects include feeling tired or drowsy the next day, memory loss, headache and problems with performance. Prescription sleeping pills can cause strange and potentially dangerous side effects. Those side effects can include dangerous allergic reactions and bizarre behaviors such as sleep eating, walking and driving, in which a person will drive a car while not fully awake and has no memory of doing so.

## SUMMARY OF THE INVENTION

There are two devices in this invention—one to use on the nose, and the other to use on the diaphragm, during practicing the process, which makes the user go to sleep, this helping to alleviate mental disorders and strokes.

Use of the nose-device and the diaphragm-device makes one breath freely and deeply. This provides more oxygen into the lungs, and into the blood-stream to alleviate problems caused by peripheral neuropathy.

## BRIEF DESCRIPTION OF THE DRAWINGS

FIG. 1 is a front-view of the nose-device when put on the nose.

FIG. 2 is a plan-view of the nose-device before it is put on the nose.

FIG. 3 is a plan-view of the diaphragm-device.

FIG. 4 is a top-view of the diaphragm-device when put on the diaphragm.

## DETAILED DESCRIPTION OF THE DRAWINGS

The user places a nose-band on his (or her) nose 10. The user also places a diaphragm-band on his (or her) diaphragm. The user lies down and closes the eyes. As a result, the user then goes to sleep 20.

In this method to induce sleep, a person is required to put on the devices, lay in bed (or sofa) and close eyes and keep them closed to cut off incoming light into the eyes and get dark-night's sleep.

Two devices are used in this method. The device to be worn on the nose is shown in FIGS. 1 and 2. It is made of a soft, flexible and elastic material. It is a band 40, configured to fit on to various nose-sizes, with self-adhesive to stay stuck on to skin and keep it comfortably on the nose while in use. The nose-band is made from rubber or equal, or any other suitable materials. The device elongates or contracts sufficiently to facilitate the user breathing air freely through the nose and deeply into the lungs. The nose-band is re-usable to help the user concentrate the mind on the device or inhalation-exhalation of the breath.

The other device used in this method, shown in FIGS. 3 and 4, is worn around the diaphragm. In FIG. 3 the diaphragm-band is shown in an open position, with the ends not joined. In FIG. 4 the diaphragm-band is shown in a closed position, with the ends joined, when it is worn around the diaphragm. It is made of a soft, flexible and elastic material. It is a band 60 configured to fit around various diaphragm-sizes, with self-adhesive ends 62, to stay stuck together and keep it comfortably on the diaphragm while in use.

The diaphragm-band is made from rubber or equal, or any other suitable material. The device elongates or contracts sufficiently to facilitate the user breathing air freely through the nose and deeply into the lungs. The diaphragm-band is re-usable to help the user concentrate the mind on the device or movement of the diaphragm while inhaling and exhaling.

In learning the method, a person can perform the following steps: The person lays in bed (or sofa) with closed-eyes, and visualizes upon a principal thought, such as on the nose-band or inhalation and exhalation of breath, until a calm mind is attained with decrease of intrusive thoughts in the mind. That practice should continue on the nose-band or inhalation and exhalation of breath or with different principal thoughts, one at a time, until one-thought which works consistently is identified. The person thinks positively in the mind and by visualizing one principal thought about any object-thing, location-spot, or action-item that exists within or without, for example the device on the nose or inhale-exhale of the breath. The person generates positive-signals in the mind by visualizing two or more principal thoughts calmly-equally at the same time, for example the device on the nose or inhalation-exhalation of the breath, and the device on the diaphragm or

**3**

movement of diaphragm, until one-set of thoughts which works consistently is identified.

It is to be understood that the present invention is not limited to the sole embodiment described above, but encompasses any and all embodiments within the scope of the following claims.

What is claimed is:

1. A method of inducing sleep, comprising the steps of:
   (a) placing on the nose of a user a nose-band with adhesive end-cups that stick to the skin;
   (b) placing a band over the diaphragm of the user, the diaphragm-band having two ends that overlap and can be joined together by self-adhesive;
   (c) wherein the user is required to lay down and close the user's eyes at the start of step and keep them closed through to cut off incoming light into the eyes and
   (d) visualizing the nose-band during inhale and exhale of breath and at the same time visualizing the band over the diaphragm to induce sleep of the user.

2. The method of inducing sleep according to claim **1**, wherein the nose-band is made of a soft, flexible and elastic material, and is configured to fit onto the nose of a user.

3. The method of inducing sleep according to claim **2**, wherein the soft, flexible and elastic material is perforated rubber.

**4**

4. The method of inducing sleep according to claim **1**, wherein the diaphragm-band is made of a soft, flexible and elastic material, and is configured to fit over the diaphragm of a user.

5. The method of inducing sleep according to claim **4**, wherein the soft, flexible and elastic material is perforated rubber.

6. The method of inducing sleep according to claim **1**, wherein the nose-band and the diaphragm-band are sufficiently elastic that the ends stay stuck and keep in position while in use for breathing air freely through the nose and deeply into the lungs.

7. A method of inducing sleep, comprising the steps of:
   (a) placing a nose band on the nose of a user;
   (b) placing a band around the torso of the user, the band having two ends that overlap and can be secured together;
   (c) wherein the user is lies down and closes the user's eyes and
   (d) visualizing the nose-band during inhale and exhale of breath and at the same time visualizing the band around the torso to induce sleep of the user.

\* \* \* \* \*

# 1. Fed. Cir's non-precedential order of Nov. 10, 2011

United States Court of Appeals for the Federal Circuit
2011-1389

**M. R. MIKKILINENI,**
Plaintiff-Appellant,
v.

**Robert Stoll, Commissioner of Patents,**
Defendant-Appellee.

------------------------------------------------------------------------------------

Appeal from the US District Court for the Eastern District of Virginia
in case no. 09cv1412, judge L.M.Brinkema.

------------------------------------------------------------------------------------

Decided: Nov. 10, 2011

---------------------------

M.R.Mikkilineni, of Washington, DC, pro se

Raymond T. Chen, Solicitor, Office of the Solicitor, US Patent and
Trademark Office of Alexandria, Virginia for the defendant-appellee.
With him on the brief were Mary L. Kelly and Scott C. Weidenfeller,
Associate Solicitors.

---------------------------------------------

Before RADER, Chief judge, LOURIE, and MOORE, Circuit Judges.

Per Curiam.
M.R.Mikkilineni appeals from the district court's denial of his motion
under FRCP 60(b)(3) requesting relief from a final judgment due to
alleged fraud by the US Patent and Trademark Office (PTO). Because
Mikkilineni fails to show any evidence of fraud, misrepresentation, or
misconduct by the PTO and merely reargues his earlier appeal of the
underlying judgment, we affirm.

This is the second appeal arising from this case and the background
is detailed in *Mikkilineni v. Stoll*, 410 Fed Appx 311 (Fed Cir 2011)

(First Appeal). To summarize, Mikkilineni applied for a patent for a "Method of Inducing Sleep" involving "concentrating upon principal thoughts to calm mind" and the use of certain devices to aid in the method. The examiner rejected the claims based on the PTO's Interim Patent Subject Matter Eligibility Examination Instructions (Interim Guidelines) that were issued to aid patent examiners in evaluating subject matter eligibility under 35 USC @101. Mikkilineni filed suit under the Administrative Procedure Act (APA) alleging that the PTO violated 5 USC @553(b)-(c) by failing to provide for notice and public comment on the Interim Guidelines. First Appeal, 410 Fed Appx at 312. We affirmed the district court's dismissal of that case. We held that the Interim Guidelines were interpretive rather than substantive and thus did not require notice and public comment under the APA. Id at 313.

Following our judgment, Mikkilineni returned to the district court with a motion under FRCP 60(b)(3) arguing that the USPTO had obtained the previous judgment based on fraud. The district court denied this motion, holding that Mikkilineni "fails to meet the clear and convincing evidence standard; instead, he merely repeats the legal arguments that he already presented." J.A 2. Further, Mikkilineni "may disagree with the defendant's legal positions, but that disagreement does not establish that a fraud was committed." Id. Mikkilineni appeals; we have jurisdiction under 28 USC @1295(a)(1).

FRCP 60(b)(3) provides:
On motion and just terms, the court may relieve a party or its legal representative from a final judgment, order or proceeding for the following reasons:
***
(3) fraud (whether previously called intrinsic or extrinsic), misrepresentation, or misconduct by an opposing party.

In reviewing a Rule 60(b) motion, we apply the law of the regional circuit. Amstar Corp. v. Envirotech Corp., 823 F.2d 1538, 1550 (Fed Cir 1987). We review the trial court's determination for an abuse of discretion. *MLC Auto., LLC v. Town of S.Pines*, 532 F.3d 269, 277 (4th Cir. 2008). A court abuses its discretion when it "has acted arbitrarily or irrationally,.. has failed to consider judicially recognized factors constraining its exercise of discretion, or when it has relied on erroneous factual or legal premises." *United States v. Hedgepath*, 418 F.3d 411, 419 (4th Cir. 2005).

Mikkilineni asserts that a number of PTO actions amount to fraud including, among other things, (1) the PTO's assertion that the correct avenue to challenge the Interim Guidelines was through a direct appeal of a final rejection, (2) the PTO's characterization of the Interim Guidelines as interpretive rather than substantive, (3) the PTO's argument that Mikkilineni asked the courts to rewrite the Interim Guidelines, (4) the PTO's factual assertion that Mikkilineni failed to comment on the Interim Guidelines when PTO voluntarily requested public comment, and (5) the PTO's final rejection of claims one day after the expiry of Mikkilineni's deadline to request Supreme Court review of the First Appeal. Mikkilineni argues that this fraud entitles him to relief from the district court's earlier judgment.

We agree with the district court that Mikkilineni fails to show any evidence of fraud. Instead, he reargues the merits of the First Appeal and accuses the PTO of fraud and misrepresentation for disagreeing with his positions. The PTO is correct that Mikkilineni is free to challenge all of the bases of rejection in a direct appeal and that is the the correct route for his complaints. The district court did not abuse its discretion in determining that Mikkilineni failed to show evidence of fraud, and thus, we affirm.
AFFIRMED

**2.** Order of April 7, 2011
IN THE UNITED STATES DISTRICT COURT FOR THE
EASTERN DISTRICT OF VIRGINIA, Alexandria Division

M. R. Mikkilineni, Plaintiff,
v.                                   1:09cv1412(LMB/JFA)
                                     Filed APR 7, 2011
Robert Stoll, Defendant.

ORDER
The pro se plaintiff M. R. Mikkilineni has filed a Motion for Relief
under Rule 60(b)(3) and Allow the Action to Proceed Under Rule
60(d)(1) based on New- Evidence [Mot. for Relief Under Rule 60(b)
(3)] [Dkt. No. 39], which this Court construes as a motion for relief
from the Court's April 30, 2010 final judgment dismissing plaintiff's
complaint with prejudice for lack of subject matter jurisdiction.1 The
Court denied a motion to reconsider the judgment on May 18, 2010.
The United States Court of Appeals for the Federal Circuit affirmed
the dismissal on November 9, 2010, and no further appeal has been
taken from that decision, which has now become final.

Under Fed. R. Civ. P. 60(b), "a court may relieve a party from a final
judgment, order or proceeding on several grounds, including: mistake,
inadvertence or surprise,- the emergence of evidence not previously
available; fraud; and any other reason that justifies relief." Power
Paragon, Inc. v. Precision Tech. USA, Inc., 2008 U.S. Dist. LEXIS
109720 (E.D. Va. Dec. 18, 2008). Without providing any evidence
to support his claim, plaintiff argues that the defendant perpetrated a
fraud on the Court in the earlier proceedings. To obtain relief under
Fed. R. Civ. P. 60(b) for fraud, the plaintiff must demonstrate through
clear and convincing evidence that the fraud adversely impacted
"the full and fair preparation or presentation of its case," Anderson
v. Cryovac, Inc., 862 F.2d 910, 923 {1st Cir. 1988). Plaintiff fails to

---

1 Plaintiff's motion also refers to Fed. R. Civ. P. 60(d)(1), which states: "Other
Powers to Grant Relief. This rule does not limit a court's power to: entertain an
independent action to relieve a party from a judgment, order, or proceeding." This
rule does not provide a separate basis for relief from final judgment. Therefore, the
Court considers this motion only under Fed. R. Civ P. 60(b).

meet the clear and convincing evidence standard; instead, he merely repeats the legal arguments that he already presented to this Court. Plaintiff may disagree with the defendant's legal positions, but that disagreement does not establish that a fraud was committed.

Moreover, the defendant's legal positions were accepted by this Court and the Federal Circuit. Accordingly, it is hereby

ORDERED that plaintiff's Motion for Relief under Rule 60(b)(3) [Dkt. No. 39], be and is DENIED.

To appeal this Order, plaintiff must file a written Notice of Appeal with the Clerk of this Court within sixty (60) days of the date of this Order.

The Clerk is directed to forward copies of this Order to plaintiff, pro se, at his address of record, and to counsel of record, and to remove the hearing on this motion from this Court's April 8, 2011 docket.

Entered this 7th day of April, 2011. Alexandria, Virginia
/s/
Leonie M. Brinkema, US judge

**3.** Fed. Cir's non-precedential order of Nov. 9, 2010
United States Court of Appeals for the Federal Circuit
2010-1362

**M. R. MIKKILINENI,**
**Plaintiff-Appellant,**
**v.**

**Robert Stoll, Commissioner of Patents,**
Defendant-Appellee.

-----------------------------------------------------------------------------------

Appeal from the US District Court for the Eastern District of Virginia
in case no. 09cv1412, judge L.M.Brinkema.

-----------------------------------------------------------------------------------

Decided: Nov. 9, 2010

-----------------------------

M.R.Mikkilineni, of Washington, DC, pro se

Raymond T. Chen, Solicitor, Office of the Solicitor, US Patent and
Trademark Office of Alexandria, Virginia for the defendant-appellee.
With him on the brief were Mary L. Kelly and Scott C. Weidenfeller,
Associate Solicitors.

---------------------------------------------

Before GAJARSA, LINN, and DYK, Circuit Judges.

Per Curiam.
M.R.Mikkilineni (Mikkilineni) appeals from a decision of the US
District Court for the Eastern District of Virginia dismissing his
claims with prejudice under FRCP 12(b)(1) and (6). *Mikkilineni v.
Stoll*, No. 09cv1412 (ED Va Apr 30,2010). We *affirm*.

Background
Mikkilineni filed a patent application which discloses and claims
"a method to fall-asleep by learning to use the process-algorithm
in the brain (to) transform brain-neurons into a different physical

state and produce melatonin and serotonin… without the use of drugs." Appellee's App A64-65. Mikkilineni's claims were rejected in a non-final rejection under 35 USC @101 as non-statutory subject matter. During a meeting with Mikkilineni and his patent attorney, the examiner explained that he was required to reject the claims as non-statutory subject matter based on the US Patent and Trademark Office's (USPTO) Interim Patent Subject Matter Eligibility Examination Instructions (Interim Guidelines).1 The Interim Guidelines provide that "purely mental processes in which thoughts or human based actions are 'changed' are not considered an eligible transformation." USPTO, Interim Examination Instructions for Evaluating Subject Matter Eligibility Under 35 USC @101 (Aug. 25, 2009), available at http://www.uspto.gov/web/offices/pac/dapp/opla/2009-08-25_interim_instructions.pdf.

The Interim Guidelines were posted on the USPTO's official website with a notice requesting public comment and indicating a deadline for receipt of comments. Though not required to do so, the USPTO also published a request for comments in the Federal Register. See Request for Comments on Interim Examination Instructions for Evaluating Patent Subject Matter Eligibility, 74 Fed Reg 47,780 (Sept 17, 2009) (Request for Comments). The Request for Comments included an explanation that the Interim Guidelines were interpretive guidance based on the USPTO's current understanding of the law, stating specifically that the "Examination Instructions do not constituted substantive rule making and hence do not have the force and effect of law." Id. The Request for Comments further advised that "rejections are and will continue to be based upon the substantive law." Id.

Mikkilineni filed a response to the Office Action and, one day later, filed suit under the Administrative Procedure Act (APA) to challenge the USPTO's Interim Guidelines, alleging that the USPTO violated 5 USC @553(b)-(c) by failing to provide notice and an opportunity for comment on interim interpretive guidance issued

---

1 The Interim Guidelines were issued by the USPTO to aid patent examiners in evaluating subject matter eligibility during the time between this court's decision in *In re Bilski*, 545 F.3d 943 (Fed Cir 2008) (en banc), and the Supreme Court's decision in *Bilski v. Kappos*, 130 S.Ct. 3218 (2010).

by the agency. Complaint, *Mikkilineni v. Stoll,* No.09cv1412 (ED Va Apr 30, 2009). The district court granted USPTO's motion to dismiss under FRCP 12(b)(1) and (6). We have jurisdiction pursuant to 28 USC @1295(a)(1).


Discussion

We review orders dismissing under Rules 12(b)(1) or (6) de novo. *Boyle v. US,* 200 F.3d 1369, 1372 (Fed Cir 2000). On appeal, Mikkilineni contends that: (1) the Interim Guidelines are substantive rules improperly promulgated without notice and comment rulemaking, and (2) the USPTO examiner improperly rejected his application. We reject both claims.

I

Under @553 of the APA, certain agency actions require prior public notice and comment. 5 USC @553. Generally speaking, "substantive" rules require notice and comment, while "interpretive" rules do not. 5 USC @553(b)(3)(A); *Lincoln v. Vigil,* 508 US 182, 195-96 (1993); *Animal Legal Defense Fund v. Quigg,* 932 F.2d 920, 927 (Fed Cir 1991). A rule is "substantive" where it causes a change in existing law or policy that affects individual rights and obligations and "interpretive" where it "merely clarifies or explains existing law or regulations." *Animal Legal Defense Fund,* 932 F.2d at 927.

Mikkilineni argues that the Interim Guidelines are substantive rules within the meaning of the APA because they substantively deprived him of his rights by requiring the Examiner to reject his claims under @101. This argument is without merit. The USPTO's Request for Comments explicitly states both (1) that the guidelines are "based on the USPTO's current understanding of the law and are believed to be fully consistent with binding precedent," and (2) that the guidelines "do not have the force and effect of law""; thus, "rejections are and will continue to be based upon substantive law." 74 Fed Reg at 47,780.

Our decision in *Animal Legal Defense Fund* is almost directly on point. See 932 F.2d at 920. In that case, the plaintiffs argued that a notice issued by the USPTO in response to the Supreme Court's decision in *Diamond v. Chakrabarty*, 447 US 303 (1980), was substantive rule making and, as a result, must be promulgated via notice and comment rulemaking. *Animal Legal Defense Fund*, 932 F.2d at 923-24. The notice, which stated "that the PTO 'now considers non-naturally occurring, non-human multicellular organisms, including animals, to be patentable subject matter within the scope of 35 USC @101," mirrored the Supreme Court's holding in *Diamond*. Id at 922-923; *see also diamond*, 447 US at 309. This court rejected the plaintiff's argument, finding that the USPTO notice was interpretive rather than substantive. *Animal Legal Defense Fund*, 932 F.2d at 931. Accordingly, we conclude that the Interim Guidelines are interpretive, rather than substantive, and are thus exempt from the notice and comment requirements of @553 of the APA. See Lincoln, 508 US at 195-96; *Animal Legal Defense Fund*, 932 F.2d at 927. As a result, the district court's dismissal under Rule 12(b)(6) was proper.

II

The district court also correctly held that it lacked jurisdiction to review the examiner's non-final rejection. Under the APA, final agency action is required before judicial review is permitted. 5 USC @704. As a general rule, two conditions must be met for agency action to be considered final under the APA: (1) "the action must mark the 'consummation' of the agency's decision making process— it must not be of a merely tentative or interlocutory nature"; and (2) "the action must be one by which 'rights or obligations have been determined,' or from which 'legal consequences will flow." *Bennett v. Spear*, 520 US 154, 177-78 (1997) (internal citations omitted).

There has been no final agency action in this case. The non-final rejection of Mikkilineni's claims did not constitute the consummation of the agency's decision making process. Mikkilineni's claims are still pending—no final rejection has been entered. All prosecution in his application has been stayed pending the outcome of this litigation. After a non-final rejection, the applicant may reply to the rejection and "the application or the patent...will be reconsidered and again examined." 37 CFR @1.112. When the examiner issues a final rejection Mikkilineni may appeal to the Board of Patent Appeals and Interferences (Board). Only after a Board decision affirming

a final rejection is judicial review available. Additionally, the non-final rejection by the examiner is not an action from which legal consequences will flow—in theory, Mikkilineni could still overcome the non-final rejection and receive a patent. As a result, the district court's dismissal under Rule 12(b)(1) was proper.
AFFIRMED

**4.** Order of April 30, 2010
IN THE UNITED STATES DISTRICRT COURT FOR THE
EASTERN DISTRICRT OF VIRGINIA, ALEXANDRIA DIVISION

M.R.Mikkilineni, Plaintiff,

v.                                   1:09cv1412(LMB/JFA)
                                     Filed APR 30 2010
Robert Stoll, Defendant.

ORDER

For the reasons stated* in open court, defendant's motion to dismiss is
Granted and plaintiff's motion to set aside USPTO's substantive rule
& enter declaratory order is Denied, and it is hereby Ordered that this
civil action be and is dismissed with Prejudice.
The clerk is directed to forward copies of this Order to plaintiff, pro
se, at his address of record, and to counsel of record, and to enter final
judgment in favor of the defendant under FRCP 58.
If the plaintiff, pro se, wishes to appeal this order, he must file a
written Notice of Appeal with the clerk of this court within sixty days
of the date of this order.
Entered this 30th day of April, 2010.

Sd/
Leonie Brinkema, US Judge

*"The reality of it is that the lawsuit that you (applicant) have filed
in this court and the motion, have no legal foundation.  As the
government has correctly pointed out, you have not yet had a final
agency action- patent has not finally been rejected... without a final
action from the agency, you really have no basis to be in this court.
The case is dismissed and your motion to set aside the substantive
rule is denied."

Copy of Adam pleadings filed in the courts

**UNITED STATES DISTRICT COURT** FOR *EASTERN DISTRICT OF VIRGINIA*

M.R.Mikkilineni
PO Box 32110
Washington, DC 20007
      Plaintiff,
v.
                          Related to No:09cv1412
                          Judge Brinkema

Robert Stoll, Commissioner for Patents
USPTO, PO Box 1450
Alexandria, Va. 22313-1450

## *Complaint*

### I. Jurisdiction:

1. Under 5 USCS § 551-3(c) & (e): Agency shall give an interested person the right to petition for the issuance, amendment, or repeal of a rule...

2. Under 5 USCS § 702 & 706(1) & (2): To the extent necessary to decision and when presented, the reviewing court shall decide all relevant questions of law, interpret constitutional and statutory provisions, and determine the meaning or applicability of the terms of an agency action... and the reviewing court shall— 702 hold agency action wrong or adversely affected or aggrieved...

706(1) order agency to take a discrete action that it is required to take...

706(2) hold agency action unlawful and set aside findings, and conclusions found to be–

(A) arbitrary, capricious, an abuse of discretion, or otherwise not in accordance with law;

3. Under 28 USCS § 2201(a): In a case of actual controversy within its jurisdiction,… any court of the United States, upon the filing of an appropriate pleading, may declare the rights and other legal relations of any interested party seeking such declaration, whether or not further relief is or could be sought.

## II.   Parties:

4.. Plaintiff M.R.Mikkilineni is a retired professional engineer and an Indian-American, reside in Washington, DC, with mailing address at PO Box 32110, Washington DC 20007.

(i)   Plaintiff is the sole-inventor of the "process" or method to induce sleep (without use of pill or drug…).

5. Defendant Robert Stoll is the Commissioner for Patents at PTO, with mailing address at P.O Box Box 1450, Alexandria, Va. 22313-1450.

**III.** *Factual* background (from *original*-Complaint):

6. Sometime in 2005-6, I perfected an idea how to activate the 'master clock' in the brain for a sleep-cycle by flipping off the 'light-switch' in the brain stem, and fall asleep instantly.

(i) In this 'process' specific-neurons in the brain (see research conducted at U of Wisconsin) gets transformed into a different state, and produce melatonin and serotonin and activates the master clock in the brain for a sleep-cycle.

(ii) The 'process' works this way- learn to generate positive-signals using specific positive-thoughts in the mind, input those signals into the brain-algorithm (the *circuits* in the brain…), and process the signals in the brain until the neurons get transformed and induce a sleep-cycle.

(iii) The 'process' tunes the brain and clears excited negative-signals generated by natural phenomena or streaming intrusive thoughts into the mind as a result of anxiety, anger, depression or mental-disorder(s).

(iv) Brain has two hemispheres and one is dominant; the two hemispheres communicate with each other, one thought at a time. Any interference from two or more thoughts in the mind, at the same instant or time, creates havoc with motor-responses in the brain, then the two hemispheres stop communicating- a split brain. That split brain causes the light switch 'flip' in the brain stem, activate the master-clock, and make brain fall-asleep; that helps cure depression or mental-disorder(s).

(v) Brain is the control center of the body; it controls thought-signals, senses, memory and function of cells-organs. Survival depends on a properly functioning brain to regulate the functions of the organs; it requires a sleep-cycle, of about 8-hours in a 24-hour day to function properly. A recent study at Harvard Medical School and University of California concludes-

*"...a lack of sleep causes the brain's emotional centers to dramatically overreact...*(with) *psychiatric disorders...* (and) *fractures the brain mechanisms that regulate key aspects of mental health... and, sleep appears to restore emotional brain's circuits...."*

(vi) The National Sleep Foundation's (NSF) sleep in America poll found that 74% of American adults experience sleep problems a few nights a week or more, 39% get less than seven hours of sleep each weeknight, and more than one in three (37%) are so sleepy during the day that it interferes with daily activities. *"1 in 10 suffers from chronic insomnia and it is estimated that sleeplessness costs the US economy $35 billions a year...."*

(vii) At this stage, science is trying to find a way to implant a new 'gene' or light switch in the brain for treating mental-disorder(s), and/or to control sleep-wake state of the brain with a flip of the light switch; but, unable to locate or 'repair' the light switch that exists in the brain stem.

(viii)  My 'process' or method is able to 'repair' the light-switch and make it work <u>without</u> an implant or use of pills or drugs.

7.  So, on **June 08, 2006** or nearly **5** years ago, I made an application for Patent (at No.11/449,519) with PTO.

(i)  If I place my process into practice or start a teaching-School, without Patent protection, the pill or drug-makers could start a parallel organization and drive me out; then, keep selling pills or drugs making money and causing *ill* health to millions of People.

(ii)  On Dec. 21, 2006, my petition is granted to make 'special' or expedite review based on my *ill*-health; on Jan. 17, 2007, examiner sent me claim rejections (non-final) under 35 USC @101, as *non-statutory subject matter*; under 35 USC @112 paras. 1-2: failing to comply with *enablement requirement* and failing to *define* the invention...

(iii)  At the suggestion of examiner, I hired a Patent-attorney, Mr.Swift, Esq.; and timely filed an amendment.
(iv)  On May 30, 2007, Mr.Swift and I met Mr.Pezzuto, examiner (supervisor of Art Unit 3714); Mr.Pezzuto's interview summary stated *"there is no agreement as the rejection under 35 USC 101 and the examiner will discuss this with in-house authorities"*.

(v)  Subsequently, Mr.Pezzuto indicated likelihood of granting Patent because my Method has 2-prongs in it, Process and Teaching.

(vi)  On Oct. 12, 2007, examiner sent a **final** claim rejection per the dictates of *in-house authority*.

8.  On **Dec. 06, 2007**, I filed my application (at No.11/999,349), as a 'continuation in part'; my application is sent to a new examiner (Art Unit 3735).

(i)  On Aug. 07, 2008, I met Mr.Gilbert, new-examiner, and explained how any one interested in the skill can be trained to use the Method for concrete-benefit. Mr.Gilbert understood it and his interview summary stated *"Mr.Mikkilineni explained that his method was not concentrating on a scene with two elements of an image at the same time, but, keep two separate elements as two separate thoughts, (and) bring them into the mind at the same time"*.

(ii)  I made it clear that a specification or a book can't teach some-one to ride a bike, or an MD-trainee do brain-Surgery, and all of us require proper training…; if books can enable an ordinary skilled to do it, there is no need of teaching-Schools.

(iii)  On June 20, 2008, examiner sent me claim rejections (non-final) under 35 USC @101, as *non-statutory subject matter*; under 35 USC @112 paras. 1-2: as failing to comply with *enablement requirement* and as being *indefinite* claim…

(iv)  On Sept. 19, 2008, I had a telephone interview with Mr.Marmor (supervisor of Art Unit 3735), and his summary says *"applicant explained… and suggested a sleep study be conducted to address the rejections… examiner explained that **the sleep study** would likely **not be useful**… that the pending method claims involve **merely mental steps** and are unpatentable and **nonstatutory**. A patent eligible process under 35 USC 101 must be tied to another statutory class, such as a particular apparatus, or **transform** underlying subject matter or material"* (Exb. 2.4).

9.  I re-hired Mr.Swift (with limited-funds I could save out of my SS); on **Oct. 27, 2008**, Mr.Swift, Esq. filed a new application (at No.12/259,285), as a 'continuation in part'.

(i)  On Sept. 21, 2009, I discovered an article published in Washington Post on *'Meditation Gives Brain a Charge…'*, a study conducted at U. of Wisconsin with help from **Dalai Lama**.

(ii)  On **Oct. 01, 2009**, examiner sent claim *rejections* (non-final) under 35 USC @101, as *inoperative and lacks utility*; under 35 USC

@112 paras. 1-2, as failing to comply with *enablement requirement* and as being *indefinite* claim…

(iii)  Examiner issued rejection under 35 USC @ 101 on Oct. 01, 2009 or after a ruling from Fed. Cir. in <u>PROMETHEUS</u> v. MAYO, 581 F.3d 1336 where the court *re-affirmed* that under 35 USC 101 Congress intended statutory subject matter to include anything under the sun that is made by man.

(iv)  Examiner issued rejection under 35 USC @ 112 on Oct. 01, 2009, knowing Fed. Cir.'s ruling of June 28, 2007 in <u>Hyatt</u> v. Dudas, 492 F.3d 1365; and, knowing Fed Cir.'s subsequent ruling on Oct. 12, 2007 in <u>ALLVOICE</u> v. NUANCE, 504 F.3d 1236.

**IV** *Relevant*-**Facts** (from *notarized* pleading filed on or about April 15, 2010)**:**

10.  On **Oct. 27, 2009**, Mr.Swift, Esq. and I met examiner Gilbert, and supervisor Marmor (Art Unit 3735); I presented that my method with 2-prongs, the process and the teaching, satisfies all the requirements of 35 USC @ 101 & 112, because the process part *transforms* brain-neurons into a different state for a specific purpose, and the teaching (or training) part *enables* one in the skill of the art *understand the bounds of my claim* and be able to use after learning  the method.

(i)  Then, Marmor gave me a copy of 11-page memorandum dated **Aug. 24, 2009** (signed by A.H.Hirshfeld) '**New Interim Patent Subject Matter Eligibility Examination Instructions**' (under 35 USC @101) which is made effective on Aug. 24, 2009.

(ii)  Gilbert and Marmor pointing to (on page 5) a sentence "***Purely mental processes in which thoughts or human based actions are 'changed' are not considered an eligible transformation***", informed me of their inability to accept my Method because of that *new* rule. And, assured me no other examiner would be able to do any better because Commissioner (Stoll) and others are aware of this *new*-rule and my Process…

(iii) On **Oct. 28, 2009**, examiner Gilbert issued an Interview Summary, a copy of which attorney Swift mailed to me on Dec. 19, 2009, which confirmed the substance of examiner's rejection of my Patent claims-

*"The examiner took the position that the process is not statutory because 'Purely mental processes in which thoughts or human based actions are "changed" are not considered an eligible transformation', page 5 of the 'Interim Examination Instructions for Evaluating Subject Matter Eligibility under 35 USC 101'".*

(iv) On **Oct. 28-29, 2009**, I promptly submitted my comments, suggestions or objections to PTO well before the deadline date of **Nov. 9, 2009** (Exb. 3.6) based on the substance of examiner's rejection or PTO's change in policy- **"affirms prior-practice of discrimination against '*mental-process*', a judicially recognized exception, which is central to the purpose of the method I invented; and, the *mental process* in my method is limited to making *neurons* (specific to brain) attain a *different-state* or reduce to an active-state in producing melatonin-serotonin for the sleep-cycle (*a particular practical application*). Sec 101"**

(v) Although the Notice advised that *"the PTO will revise the* (Interim Guidance) *instructions as appropriate based on comments received"*, I did <u>not</u> receive any response to my comments from PTO other than a suggestion (on phone…) *"take an appeal to the Board"*.

(vi) PTO did <u>not</u> notify me (or my patent-attorney) on-

(1) Its *"..consideration of the relevant matter presented"* by me or whether it *"incorporate(d) in the rule adopted* (which affected my rights) *a concise general statement of the basis and purpose"* as required under @ 553(c); and,

(2) Whether it *"..gave an interested person* (in my case…) *the right to petition for the issuance, amendment, or repeal of a rule"* as required under @ 553(e).

(vii)  PTO's failure to *repeal* the *new* rule has affected my rights. PTO's misuse of *new* rule in rejecting my patent is arbitrary, capricious, an abuse of discretion, or otherwise not in accordance with law; contrary to constitutional right, power, privilege, or immunity; in excess of statutory jurisdiction, authority, or limitations; and without observance of procedure required by law [under @551-3(c) & (e) and 702, 706(1) & (2)].

(viii)  PTO thru examiner Gilbert took that position '*in excess of statutory authority*' knowing 35 USC 101 (US Congress..) did not provide for PTO's '*at-will rejection* by *taking any position under the Sun*', disregarding the evidence in the record-

(1)  "..**present invention can produce a useful, tangible, and concrete result... the split brain transforms brain-neurons into a different-physical state to flip off the light switch in the brain-stem. The brain having been repaired and transformed produces melatonin...**", and

(2)  Study at U. of Wisconsin "**meditation not only changes the working of the brain in the short term, but also quite possibly produces permanent changes...**"

11.  PTO and its "*in-house authority*" discriminated against me, or my method for nearly **5** years in favor of the pill or the drug-makers, and abused discretion; then, came up with a *new* rule in **Aug. 2009**, and upon my timely comments PTO did <u>not</u> amend or repeal that *new*-rule under 5 USCS § 553(e).

**V** *New*-**evidence** of *fraud or misrepresentations*:

12.  PTO's *misrepresentations* on **04/30/2010** (see court-transcript).

(i)  PTO (on p.3, L24-5): "*when the examiner enters final rejections,... he'll have the ability to appeal at that time*". PTO knew *final* rejection and appeal is <u>not</u> the issue in my Complaint filed under 5 USC @553(c) & (e) and 706 (Complaint at para 10 &

11)- I asserted claim for denial of my rights under the *new* rule, and requested this court to decide whether PTO's *new*-rule is substantive.

(ii) PTO (on p.4, L23-4): *"PTO made very clear that because it is an interpretive rule, it's not substantive rule making,"*. PTO knew under the guise of interpretive rules it included this *new* rule, a *substantive* rule with an intent to deprive my rights under 5 USC @531-3(c) & (e) and 702, 706(1) & (2), and upon my timely comments it did <u>not</u> repeal the *new* rule (Complaint at para 10 & 11).

(iii) PTO (on p.5, L7-10 & L15-7): *"That's correct"* no article III court has the ability to rewrite the interpretive rules of PTO… *"To the extent that the APA even applied to this interpretive guidance, that would be in our view the limits of this court's authority"*. PTO knew my claim under 5 USC @553(c ) & (e) and 706 is not *"to rewrite the interpretive rules"*, but *"to set aside that one new rule"*, which PTO has used or misused against me for nearly 5-years, and deprived my rights.

(iv) PTO (on p.5, L19-25): *"Fed. Cir. has said very clearly that it has the authority to tell the PTO that its interpretive guidance is wrong… on the merits, correct. That when it receives an appeal from the Patent Board of a rejection of a particular patent application from an applicant like Mikkilineni,.."*. PTO knew this court has jurisdiction under 5 USC @553(c) & (e) and 706 to tell the PTO its *new* rule is wrong, and Mikkilineni need not wait for Patent Board rejection of appeal under 35 USC @101 etc. since these two statutes are different.

(v) PTO (on p.7, L1-3): *"there would be no standing for an individual…unless there was some reasonable expectation that it would be applied against them in a detrimental way,"*. PTO knew it applied the *new* rule against me in a detrimental way for nearly 4 years by then.

(vi) PTO in its pleadings filed in this court (and in Fed. Cir.) "… *Mikkilineni had an opportunity to comment on the Interim guidelines- both before and after the examiner issued an initial rejection of Mikkilineni's claims on October 27, 2009- but failed to do so undermines his current claim that the PTO deprived him of any rights under the APA*". PTO knew I timely filed comments to the Notices and PTO did <u>not</u> act or repeal the new rule (see attached Exb.3.6 & 4.3).

13. PTO's (above) willful *misrepresentations* caused this court to

conclude (p.7, L12-24):

*"the reality of it is that the lawsuit.. filed in this court and the motion..., have no legal foundation. As the government has correctly pointed out,.. not yet had a final agency action... patent has not finally been rejected... without a final action from the agency, .. no basis to be in this court.. motion to set aside the substantive rule is denied"*(p.9, L6-8).

(i)  This court did so without discovery or allowing me present evidence; and the court did <u>not</u> decide- whether the *new* rule is interpretive or substantive. Also, the court bypassed the issue I raised- whether PTO has '*failed to take a discrete action*', which it is required to take upon receiving my timely comments, to repeal the *new* rule.

(ii)  The court on April 30, 2010 (order-1) *"dismissed with prejudice"* my Complaint.

(iii)  On December 22, 2010, Fed. Cir. *denied* my appeal (order-2) affirming order of this court on the issue- *"no basis to be in this court"* (for lack of jurisdiction); in doing so, Fed. Cir. went ahead to approve PTO's *new* rule as interpretive in the absence of jurisdiction in deciding- 'whether PTO's *new* rule is interpretive'- because, this court did <u>not</u> reach to that issue when it dismissed my complaint for lack of jurisdiction. Therefore, under our '*rule of law*', Fed. Cir.'s opinion approving of PTO's *new* rule is <u>*void*</u>.

(iv)  PTO, on March 23, 2011- one day after expiry of 90-day time to petition USSC- entered a '*final* rejection' of patent. In doing so, it freely used the *new* rule- *"purely mental process in which thoughts or human actions are changed is not considered patentable..."*- at least *five* times in rejecting evidence in my affidavit (Exb. 3.7.1) and the patent under @101 (see final-1). In conclusion PTO's *final* rejection says-

*"the examiner agrees that thoughts produce brain-neuron changes in the brain, however, these transformations are not considered an eligible transformation.."*

(v) PTO refused to repeal its *new* rule for the second time disregarding my comments I filed timely on Aug. 05, 2010 (see Exb. 4.3) with PTO, in response to its latest Notice of '*Interim Bilski Guidance*'. In *Bilski* the Supreme Court said-

*"concerns about attempts to call any form of human activity a process can be met by making sure the claim meets the requirement of @101"*

And, Supreme Court did <u>not</u> rule that transformation of brain-neurons thru '*mental process*' is <u>not</u> patentable- as PTO's *new* rule says without any basis...

(vi) Thus, PTO continued to discriminate my process for nearly 5-years, *first* through the '*in-house authority*', then, put into effect a *new* rule, to make my compliance essentially impossible, and substantively deprived my rights under 5 USC @ 551-3(c) & (e) and 702, 706(1) & (2).

Respectfully,

M.R.Mikkilineni
PO Box 32110
Washington, DC 20007

I certify that I hand delivered a copy of this pleading on March 28, 2011 to the office of US attorney ED of Va. at-

D C Barghaan, Esq.
Assist. US attorney
2100 Jamieson Ave.
Alexandria, Va. 22314

**UNITED STATES DISTRICT COURT** FOR *EASTREN DISTRICT OF VARGINIA*

M.R.Mikkilineni
PO Box 32110
Washington, DC 20007
      Plaintiff,
v.                                No:09cv1412
                                    Judge Brinkema
Robert Stoll, Commissioner for Patents

**Plaintiff's *Motion* to set aside** USPTO's ***Substantive***-rule & enter a declaratory-order

Dear Honorable Judge:

On the basis of the relevant-*facts* and the *law* cited in my pleading 'response-memorandum of law' filed on this day, I request the court to enter an order under 5 USC @ 706(2) to set aside USPTO's substantive rule on page 5 in the 'Interim Guidance' made effective on August 24, 2009 that *"Purely mental processes in which thoughts or human based actions are 'changed' are not considered an eligible transformation"*, as it is arbitrary, capricious, an abuse of discretion and contrary to constitutional right, privilege; and under 28 USC @ 2201(a) declare that the one-sentence new-rule in the 'Interim Guidance' is being *applied against this applicant in a way that makes his compliance essentially impossible and substantively deprives his right*, therefore, in the interest of Public, expedite review of his pending Patent-application by an examiner with expertise in transformation of brain-neurons or Mr.Pezzuto with bio-medical expertise is positive in 2007 (until the in-house authority dictates...).

In <u>Commonwealth</u> v. US, 2009 US Dist. LEXIS 110293, judge Friedman of USDC/DC said-

*"To justify the issuance of (a preliminary) injunction, the (plaintiff) must show that unless the rule is enjoined, the (plaintiff) is likely to experience not just some injury, but irreparable harm that cannot be cured by ultimate success on the merits in this case. See <u>Wisc. Gas</u>, 758 F.2d 669... Further, the (plaintiff) must show that the alleged*

*harm will directly result from the action which (plaintiff) seeks to enjoin... The notice-and-comment provisions of the APA are designed-(1) to ensure that agency regulations are tested via exposure to diverse public comment, (2) to ensure fairness to affected parties, and (3) to give affected parties an opportunity to develop evidence in the record to support their objections to the rule and thereby enhance the quality of judicial review. Environmental, 425 F.3d 992.*

*As the D.C. Circuit has pointed out, Sec. 553 is designed to ensure that affected parties have an opportunity to participate in and influence agency decision making at an early stage, when the agency is more likely to give real consideration to alternative ideas. New Jersey, 626 F.2d 1038. And the APA requires that comments submitted by members of the public be considered (not simply received) by the agency. [P]ermitting the submission of views after the effective date of a regulation is no substitute for the right of interested persons to make their views known to the agency in time to influence the rule making process in a meaningful way. American Fed'n of Govt. Emp., 655 F.2d at 1158. If the Interim... Rule is not enjoined prior to its effective date the (plaintiff) will never have an equivalent opportunity to influence the Rule's contents. The public interest is served when administrative agencies comply with their obligations under the APA. 626 F.2d at 1045 ("It is now a commonplace that notice-and-comment rule-making is a primary method of assuring that an agency's decisions will be informed and responsive)".*

In my case the harm done to the Public interest is irreparable and that cannot be cured by ultimate success on the merits in this case; and, the harm will continue from this action if the substantive rule, made effective on August 24, 2009 prior to notice-and-comment provisions of the APA are designed to protect, is not set aside because the time for a (preliminary) injunction has passed. Therefore, the court should enter an order under 5 USC @ 706(2) and set aside USPTO's substantive rule on page 5 in the 'Interim Guidance' which is made effective on August 24, 2009.

In Tierney, 718 F.2d 231 (DC Cir.) said-
*"Given that the IRS intends to release this information to SSA, the controversy is of 'sufficient immediacy' to warrant issuance of a*

*declaratory judgment. <u>Maryland</u>, 312 US 270. <u>Aetna</u>, 300 US 227
(the controversy must be "real and substantial"). Moreover, as this
court said in <u>President</u>, 627 F.2d 353 n.76 (a declaratory judgment
will ordinarily be granted only when it will either 'serve a useful
purpose in clarifying the legal relations in issue' or 'terminate and
afford relief from the uncertainty, insecurity, and controversy giving
rise to the proceeding'). A declaratory judgment here not only will put
an end to the uncertainty and insecurity faced by the appellants, but
also inform the government that release of tax information on Benefits
recipients may subject it to millions of dollars in damages...
Appellees suggest that declaratory relief is precluded because
appellants failed to show irreparable harm. We disagree. Although a
party must demonstrate irreparable injury before obtaining injunctive
relief, such a showing is not necessary for the issuance of a declaratory
judgment. <u>Steffel</u>, 415 US 452. Nor is declaratory relief unavailable
because an alternative remedy (revocation of consent) was available
to appellants. The Federal Rules of Civil Procedure expressly provide
that 'the existence of another adequate remedy does not preclude a
judgment for declaratory relief in cases where it is appropriate'. FRCP
57. Indeed, as the Advisory Committee explained, 'declaratory relief is
alternative or cumulative and not exclusive or extraordinary. . . . The
fact that another remedy would be equally effective affords no ground
for declining declaratory relief'..."*

Therefore, under 28 USC @ 2201(a) the court should declare
that the one-sentence new-rule in the 'Interim Guidance'
that was *applied against this applicant in a way to make his
compliance essentially impossible and substantively deprived
his right*, hence, in the interest of the Public, expedite review of
his pending Patent-application by an examiner with expertise in
transformation of brain-neurons or Mr.Pezzuto with bio-medical
expertise who is positive in 2007 (until the in-house authority
dictates...).

Respectfully,

M.R.Mikkilineni
PO Box 32110
Washington, DC 20007

I certify that I hand delivered a copy of this pleading on April 15,
2010 to the office of US attorney ED of Va. at-
Mr.DC Barghaan, Esq. Assist. US attorney
2100 Jamieson Ave. Alexandria, Va. 22314

**UNITED STATES DISTRICT COURT** FOR *EASTREN DISTRICT OF VARGINIA*

M.R.Mikkilineni
       Plaintiff,

v.                                   No:09cv1412

                                           Judge Brinkema

Robert Stoll, Commissioner for Patents

**Plaintiff's *Memorandum of law* in support of his Motion** & *Response* to Defendant's *Motion to Dismiss*

Dear Honorable Judge:
I submit memorandum of law in support of my motion to set aside USPTO's substantive rule made effective on August 24, 2009, and a response to defendants' motion to dismiss. I state summary of relevant-*facts* (notarized below), and cite relevant-*law* (in the *words* of the learned judges) in support of my claim (based on the alleged-*facts* in my Complaint), and in support of this court's jurisdiction under APA (I tried to find an attorney; but, no one wants to go against USPTO due to conflict of interest):

Relevant-*facts*:

1. My claim under APA is based upon 'failure to act' or repeal of defendants' wrongful-acts.

i. On **October 28, 2009**, examiner Gilbert (Art Unit 3735) issued an Interview Summary (Exhibit 3.7), a copy of which attorney Swift mailed to me on **December 19, 2009**, which confirmed the substance of examiner's rejection of my Patent claims-

*"The examiner took the position that the process is not statutory because '**Purely mental processes in which thoughts or human based actions are "changed" are not considered an eligible transformation**', page 5 of the 'Interim Examination Instructions for Evaluating Subject Matter Eligibility under 35 USC 101'".*

ii.  At the Interview on October 27, 2009, examiner gave me a copy of the document 'Interim Examination Instructions for Evaluating Subject Matter Eligibility under 35 USC 101' (hereafter called 'Interim Guidance') which is made **effective on August 24, 2009** (Exhibit 3.5); and, he pointed out to me on page 5 that-

'*Purely mental processes in which thoughts or human based actions are "changed" are not considered an eligible transformation*'.

iii.  Examiner affirmed his rejection on the basis of this Interim Guidance, and expressed his inability to do any better on my application or no other examiner can either; I thanked the examiner and left.

iv.  Until I received defendants' motion to dismiss on or about March 31, 2010, I am not aware of USPTO's publication of a Notice (Exhibit 3.5.1) under @ 553(c) on this 'Interim Guidance...'; and, no one informed me of that either at the Interview on October 27, 2009, or at any time before or after.

v.  On October 28 and 29, 2009, I promptly submitted my comments, suggestions or objections (Exhibit 3.6) based on the substance of examiner's rejection based on USPTO's change in policy-

That it **"affirms prior-practice of discrimination against '*mental-process*', a judicially recognized exception, which is central to the purpose of the method I invented; and, the *mental process* in my method is limited to making *neurons* (specific to brain) attain a *different-state* or reduce to an active-state in producing melatonin-serotonin for the sleep-cycle (*a particular practical application*). Sec 101"**

vi.  I submitted my comments by facsimile to 571 273 0125 marked to the attention of the Commissioner on **October 28 and 29, 2009**, well before the deadline date of **November 9, 2009** (Exhibit 3.5.1).

vii.  Although the Notice advised that "*the USPTO will revise the* (Interim Guidance) *instructions as appropriate based on comments received*", I did <u>not</u> receive any response to my comments from the Commissioner other than a suggestion (on phone… as if the final-rejection is on the way) *"take an appeal to the Board"* (Exhibit 3.6).

viii.  USPTO did <u>not</u> notify me (or my Patent-attorney) on-
(1) Its *"..consideration of the relevant matter presented"* by me or whether it *"incorporate(d) in the rule adopted* (which affected my rights) *a concise general statement of the basis and purpose"* as required under @ 553(c); and,
(2)  Whether its *"required publication or service of substantive rule is made not less than 30 days before effective date"* under @ 553(d); and,
(3)  Whether it *"..gave an interested person* (in my case…) *the right to petition for the issuance, amendment, or repeal of a rule"* as required under @ 553(e).

ix. USPTO's failure-

(1)  to notify me (see at viii) of its change in policy or repeal of the rule which affected my rights under @ 553,
(2) to act on my Patent-application (Exhibit 5 on p.2/6) despite a timely response on December 23, 2009 (Exhibit 3.7.1) to examiner's rejections, is arbitrary, capricious, an abuse of discretion, or otherwise not in accordance with law; contrary to constitutional right, power, privilege, or immunity; in excess of statutory jurisdiction, authority, or limitations; and without observance of procedure required by law, under @ 706(2)(A), (B), (C), (D).

x.  On October 27, 2008, attorney Swift re-filed my Patent-application at No.12/259,285, a 2nd continuation-in-part (originally I filed for Patent on June 8, 2006, nearly 4 years ago…), per examiner Marmor's suggestion on September 24, 2008 (Exhibit 2.4.1) and his rejection that *"sleep study* (as) *likely not be useful"* because *"pending method claims involve merely mental steps and are un-patentable and non-statutory"* (Exhibit 2.4).

xi.  On September 26, 2009 (a year later…), examiner Gilbert's non-final action (Exhibit 3.4 on p.4-5) said-

Claim Rejections- 35 USC @ 101- *"Claims 1-20 are rejected under 35 USC 101 because the disclosed invention is inoperative and therefore lacks utility... In the instant case the process functions to change the processing of the brain. However it is examiner's position that changing the processing in the brain does not transform the brain... The activity caused by the method, 'cause the brain to produce melatonin' and 'helping the brain produce serotonin' are natural functions of the brain and therefore the brain has not been transformed only initiated to perform a function the brain normally performs. Therefore the claim is not directed to statutory subject matter"*.

xii. USPTO thru examiner Gilbert took that position '*in excess of statutory authority*' knowing 35 USC 101 (or Congress..) did not provide for USPTO's '*at-will rejection* by *taking any position under the Sun*', discarding the facts or evidence that stated-

(1) The fact in my application (Exhibit 3.1 on p.23-4) "..**present invention can produce a useful, tangible, and concrete result... the split brain transforms brain-neurons into a different-physical state to flip off the light switch in the brain-stem. The brain having been repaired and transformed produces melatonin...**", and
(2) The evidence or finding from a study at U. of Wisconsin (Exhibit 3.3) "**meditation not only changes the working of the brain in the short term, but also quite possibly produces permanent changes...**"

xiii. In 2009, examiner Gilbert's act in rejecting my Patent claims is identical to that of a 'trainee or junior-examiner' in 2007 (working under Mr.Pezzuto, Art Unit 3714) who acted under the dictates of an "*in-house authority*" (Exhibit 1.3); the only difference is the dictates in 2006-9 came in the absence of an 'Interim Guidance..', and by August 24, 2009, USPTO could create a change in policy to help justify the old and new dictates using or misusing <u>Biliski</u>...(see Relevant-*law*).

xiv. As of February 2008, Commissioner's office (Mr.Wu and Ms.Harrison) advised me that Mr.Pezzuto (of Art Unit 3714) has agreed to be the examiner on my application for Patent (in the second-round…); but, in mid-April 2008, I am told my application is sent to Mr.Marmor (of Art Unit 3735) and Mr.Gilbert, electrical engineer, is the examiner, **not a bio-medical expert per my request** (Exhibit 2.1.1).

xv.  On August 7, 2008, I met Mr.Gilbert, explained my Method, answered questions, and on August 19, 2008, I filed my summary of minutes (Exhibit 2.3.1); Mr.Gilbert advised that a patent-attorney (which he suggested I hire) would be able to take care of my questions on his non-final rejections of 06/20/2008 (Exhibit 2.3). See at x.

xvi.  Based on the facts known to me as of December 9, 2009, I originally commenced this action in USDC/DC at No.09-2417; on 12/21/09, judge of USDC/DC dismissed my action as the *"venue in this case lies in the ED of Virginia and not with this court"* (Exhibit 4).

xvii.  On December 24, 2009, I re-filed the same complaint with an application seeking leave to file.. in this court at No.09cv1412; thereafter, I contacted USPTO in an attempt to settle this matter amicably…promptly in the interest of the Public (Exhibit 5).

Relevant-*law*:

2.  This court has the subject matter jurisdiction in the matter under APA, and the alleged facts state a *'plausible'* claim for relief when viewed with *'judicial experience and common sense'*, as suggested by the defendant (on p.11)

i.  In Cooper, 536 F.3d 1330 (2008) Fed Cir. said-

*"We have also previously held that 35 USC @ 2(b)(2) does not authorize the Patent Office to issue "substantive" rules. See Merck, 80 F.3d 1543. "A rule is 'substantive' when it 'effects a change in existing law or policy' which 'affect[s] individual rights and obligations.'"* Animal, *932 F.2d at 927. "In contrast, a rule which merely clarifies or explains existing law or regulations is 'interpretative."*

And, in <u>Tafas</u>, 559 F.3d 1345 (2009), Fed. Cir. (*en banc*) analyzed the distinction between '*substantive*', procedural or '*interpretive*' rule-making by USPTO, and said-

"*While the text of the rules sets forth a facially reasonable procedural requirement, we are mindful of the possibility that the USPTO may in some cases attempt to apply the rules in a way that makes compliance essentially impossible and substantively deprives applicants of their rights. In such cases, judicial review will be available under* <u>5 USC @ 706</u>". In <u>Animal</u>, 932 F.2d 920 "*To establish standing to sue, a party must, at an irreducible minimum, show* (1) *that he personally has suffered some actual or threatened injury as a result of the putatively illegal conduct* (personal injury), (2) *that the injury fairly can be traced to the challenged action* (causation), *and* (3) *that the injury is likely to be redressed by a favorable decision* (effective relief). *In addition to these requirements, standing is further limited to those parties within the "zone of interests" a particular statute addresses*" (35 USC @ 101...)

That's precisely what USPTO did here using the exception under @ 553(b)(A) made effective on **August 24, 2009** an Interim Guidance... that contained at least **one-*substantive* rule to apply in a way that makes my compliance essentially impossible and substantively deprives my right.** So, in this case *judicial review will be available under* <u>5 USC @ 706</u>, because under the guise of an '*interpretive*' rulemaking USPTO effectively put out an Interim Guidance that included a '*substantive*' rule-

"***Purely mental processes in which thoughts or human based actions are 'changed' are not considered an eligible transformation***".

<u>No</u> court in the land has <u>ever</u> said "*mental processes in which thoughts or human based action*-changes.. *are not considered an eligible transformation*"; USPTO's *in-house authority* simply made this up...as if they can take '*any position under the Sun...*'

This is a change in the existing law or policy as it impermissibly substantive, inconsistent with law, arbitrary and capricious, incomprehensibly vague, impermissibly retroactive, and procedurally defective, and affects my individual rights and obligations under <u>Bilski</u>.

ii.  In <u>Bilski</u>, 545 F.3d 943 (2008), Fed Cir. (*en banc*) analyzed whether a claim reciting *mental process* is drawn to patent-eligible subject matter under 35 USC @ 101, an issue of law, and (in judges' own words) said-

"*..we address a possible misunderstanding of our decision in <u>Comiskey</u>. Some may suggest that <u>Comiskey</u> implicitly applied a new @ 101 test that bars any claim reciting a mental process that lacks significant "physical steps." We did not so hold, nor did we announce any new test at all in <u>Comiskey</u>. Rather, we simply recognized that the Supreme Court has held that mental processes, like fundamental principles, are excluded by @ 101 because "'[p]henomena of nature, though just discovered, mental processes, and abstract intellectual concepts . . . are the basic tools of scientific and technological work.'" <u>Comiskey</u>, 499 US at 1377... Because those claims failed the machine-or-transformation test, we held that they were drawn solely to a fundamental principle, the mental process of arbitrating a dispute, and were thus not patent-eligible under @ 101.*
*... when the claim at issue recites fundamental principles other than mathematical algorithms... the proper inquiry under @ 101 is not whether the process claim recites sufficient "physical steps," but rather whether the claim meets the machine-or-transformation test. As a result, even a claim that recites "physical steps" but neither recites a particular machine or apparatus, nor transforms any article into a different state or thing, is not drawn to patent-eligible subject matter. Conversely, a claim that purportedly lacks any "physical steps" but is still tied to a machine or achieves an eligible transformation passes muster under @ 101*".

Fed Cir. in conclusion, also said- "*Of course, a claimed process wherein all of the process steps may be performed entirely in the human mind is obviously not tied to any machine and **does not*** *transform any article into a different state or thing. As a result, it would not be patent-eligible under @ 101".*

By that Fed Cir. can only mean **if** *"…process steps performed entirely in the human mind **does not transform** any article* (or substance) *into a different state"* **it would not be patent-eligible** under @ 101; but, per USPTO **if "mental processes in which thoughts or human based actions** (cause) **changes,** (such changes) **are not considered an eligible transformation".** Clearly, this is a new-law or change in the rule or policy, a *substantive* change, and <u>Bilski</u> or the Congress did not give that power to USPTO. It simply assumed that power and created the law or rule on its own using or misusing <u>Bilski</u> to discriminate my method which is based on '*mental process*'. After losing four years in trying to persuade USPTO to issue Patent, now, it appears I have to spend years in appeals if I can at 71 and being a recovered *leukemia* patient…

iii. In <u>Chrysler</u>, 441 US 281, Supreme Court said-
*"Section 10 (a) of the APA, <u>5 USC 553</u>, provides that "[a] person suffering legal wrong because of agency action, or adversely affected or aggrieved by agency action . . . , is entitled to judicial review thereof. <u>5 USC 702</u>. Two exceptions to this general rule of reviewability are set out in § 10. Review is not available where "statutes preclude judicial review" or where "agency action is committed to agency discretion by law. <u>5 USC 701(a)(1), (2)</u>. Section 4 of the APA, specifies that an agency shall afford interested persons general notice of proposed rulemaking and an opportunity to comment before a substantive rule is promulgated. In order to have the force and effect of law the promulgation of agency regulations must conform with any procedural requirements imposed by Congress, for agency discretion is limited not only by substantive, statutory grants of authority, but also by the procedural requirements which assure fairness and mature consideration of rules of general application. That an agency regulation is "substantive," does not by itself give it the "force and effect of law." The legislative power of the United States is vested in the Congress, and the exercise of quasi-legislative authority by*

*governmental departments and agencies must be rooted in a grant*
*of such power by the Congress and subject to limitations which that*
*body imposes. In order for a regulation to have the force and effect*
*of law, it must have certain substantive characteristics and be the*
*product of certain procedural requisites. The pertinent provisions*
*of § 10 (e) of the APA,* 5 USC 706, *state that a reviewing court*
*shall, (2) hold unlawful and set aside agency action, findings, and*
*conclusions found to be-*
*(A) arbitrary, capricious, an abuse of discretion, or otherwise not in*
*accordance with law;*
*. . . .*

*(F) unwarranted by the facts to the extent that the facts are subject to*
*trial de novo by the reviewing court.*
5 USC 552(a)(4)(B) *gives federal district courts jurisdiction to*
*enjoin the agency from withholding agency records and to order*
*the production of any agency records improperly withheld from the*
*complainant.*

On the issue of two-exceptions to the general rule of reviewability
(1) the statute involved here does not preclude judicial review, or (2)
USPTO's action in making substantive change in the rule or policy is
not committed to its discretion under APA.

In Norton, 542 US 55, Supreme Court said-
*"The Administrative Procedure Act (APA) authorizes suit by a*
*person suffering legal wrong because of agency action, or adversely*
*affected or aggrieved by agency action within the meaning of a*
*relevant statute.* 5 USC 702. *Where no other statute provides a*
*private right of action, the agency action complained of must be*
*final agency action.* 5 USC 704. *Agency action is defined in* 5 USC
551(13) *to include **the whole or a part of an agency rule**, order,*
*license, sanction, relief, **or the equivalent or denial thereof, or***
***failure to act**. The APA provides relief for a failure to act in* 5 USC
706(1): *The reviewing court shall compel agency action unlawfully*
*withheld or unreasonably delayed.*

*The provisions of* 5 USC 702, 704, *and* 706(1) *all insist upon an "agency action" either as **the action complained of or as the action to be compelled**. The definition of that term begins with a list of five categories of decisions made or outcomes implemented by an agency: **agency rule**, order, license, sanction, or relief.* 5 USC 551(13). *All of those categories **involve circumscribed, discrete agency actions**, as their definitions make clear: an agency **statement of future effect designed to implement, interpret, or prescribe law or policy** (rule); a final disposition in a matter other than rule making (order); a permit or other form of permission (license); a prohibition or taking of other compulsory or restrictive action (sanction); or a grant of money, assistance, license, authority, etc., or recognition of a claim, right, immunity, etc., or taking of other action on the application or petition of, and beneficial to, a person (relief).* 5 USC 551(4), (6), (8), (10), (11).

*The terms following the five categories of agency action set forth in* 5 USC 551(13) *are not defined in the Administrative Procedure Act: or the equivalent or denial thereof, or failure to act. But an "equivalent thereof" must also be discrete (or it would not be equivalent), and a "denial thereof" must be the denial of a discrete listed action (and perhaps denial of a discrete equivalent). The final term in the definition set forth in* 5 USC 551(13), *"**failure to act**," is properly understood **as a failure to take an agency action**; that is, a failure to take one of the agency actions (including their equivalents) earlier defined in* 551(13). *For purposes of* 5 USC 551(a), *a failure to act is not the same thing as a denial. The latter is the agency's act of saying no to a request; the former is **simply the omission of an action without formally rejecting a request**, for example, the failure to promulgate a rule or take some decision by a statutory deadline. The important point is that a "failure to act" is properly understood to be limited, as are the other items in* 551(13), *to **a discrete action**. The only agency action that can be compelled under the Administrative Procedure Act is action legally required.*

*A claim under* 5 USC 706(1) *can proceed only where a plaintiff **asserts that an agency failed to take a discrete agency action that it is required to take… Unless and until the (agency act) is amended, such actions can be set aside as contrary to law pursuant to** 5 USC 706(2)".

In my case, USPTO clearly failed to take discrete action which it is required to take as stated under Relevant-*facts* at viii & ix.

And, in <u>Commonwealth</u> v. US, 2009 US Dist. LEXIS 110293, judge Friedman of USDC/DC said-

*"A party experiences actionable harm when "depriv[ed] of a procedural protection to which he is entitled" under the APA.* <u>Sugar Cane Growers,</u>

289 F.3d 89. *If such were not the case, "*<u>sec. 553</u>* would be a dead letter." If defendants have in fact violated the APA's notice-and-comment provisions, then, there is no question that the (plaintiff) will be injured by the implementation of the Interim... Rule.*

<u>Response to defendant-*Argument*</u>:

3. My response is provided to the relevant issues raised by the defendant; and no response is required on the other Argument or law cited by defendant (on p.9-20) as it is not relevant to APA.

i. "Plaintiff's method does not constitute patentable subject matter under 35 USC 101, as interpreted by Fed. Cir. in <u>Biliski</u>,... which allows Plaintiff to tender a response in an effort to persuade the examiner to issue a patent... Plaintiff primarily takes issue with a guidance document USPTO issued to assist its examiners in understanding the courts' interpretation of @ 101.. in <u>Biliski</u>, but before the Supreme Court's decision in the same case" (see defendant on p.1-2).

<u>Response</u>: As stated previously, USPTO's use or misuse of <u>Biliski</u> is the root cause here. Fed Cir.'s given reasons for denial of a patent in <u>Biliski</u> or the Supreme Court's expected decision (later in 2010) in that case would not change the law applicable to my 'method' because-

My 'method' encompasses an **exception** recognized by the Supreme Court in the use of *"laws of nature, natural phenomena,* [or] *abstract* *ideas.*" <u>Diehr</u>, 450 US 175. The true issue then is whether I am seeking to claim a fundamental principle (means "*laws of nature, natural phenomena, and abstract idea*") or a *mental process*. The answer is no, I am not. So, the underlying legal question is what test governs the courts as to whether my claim to a process is patentable under @ 101 or, conversely, is my claim drawn to unpatentable subject matter *because it claims only a fundamental principle.*

In my 'method' human-**brain** is a physical object, and the **neurons** in the brain, a **substance**, that *transforms* into a *different state* in the process.

<u>Bilski's</u> claim is denied for a reason, and whether or not the Supreme Court affirms that decision will not change the '*machine* or *transformation*' test that the Supreme Court approved earlier. (USPTO to look for a pretext under Biliski is no-different from its position under the Sun for 4-Yrs.)

Fed Cir. in <u>Bilski</u> answered that (in judges' own words)-
"*The Supreme Court in <u>Diehr</u> at 187, declared that while a claim drawn to a fundamental principle is unpatentable, "an application of a law of nature or mathematical formula to a known structure or process may well be deserving of patent protection." <u>Mackay Radio</u>, 306 US 86 ("While a scientific truth, or the mathematical expression of it, is not a patentable invention, a novel and useful structure created with the aid of knowledge of scientific truth may be"). The Court in <u>Diehr</u> thus drew a distinction between those claims that "seek to pre-empt the use of" a fundamental principle, on the one hand, and claims that seek only to foreclose others from using a particular "application" of that fundamental principle, on the other. Patents, by definition, grant the power to exclude others from practicing that which the patent claims. <u>Diehr</u> can be understood to suggest that whether a claim is drawn only to a fundamental principle is essentially an inquiry into the scope of that exclusion; i.e., whether the effect of allowing the claim would be to allow the patentee to pre-empt substantially all uses of that fundamental principle. If so, the claim is not drawn to patent-eligible subject matter.*"

*The Supreme Court last addressed this issue in 1981 in <u>Diehr</u>,*
*which concerned a patent application seeking to claim a process for*
*producing cured synthetic rubber products. <u>Diehr</u>, 450 US at 177.*
*The claimed process took temperature readings during cure and used*
*a mathematical algorithm, the Arrhenius equation, to calculate the*
*time when curing would be complete. Noting that a mathematical*
*algorithm alone is unpatentable because mathematical relationships*
*are akin to a law of nature, the Court nevertheless held that the*
*claimed process was patent-eligible subject matter, stating: [The*
*inventors] do not seek to patent a mathematical formula (identifies*
*abstract idea or law of nature). Instead, they seek patent protection*
*for a process of curing synthetic rubber. Their process admittedly*
*employs a well-known mathematical equation, but they do not*
*seek to pre-empt the use of that equation. Rather, they seek only to*
*foreclose from others the use of that equation in conjunction with*
*all of the other steps in their claimed process. Id at 187. The Court*
*declared that while a claim drawn to a fundamental principle is*
*unpatentable, "an application of a law of nature or mathematical*
*formula to a known structure or process may well be deserving of*
*patent protection." See also <u>Mackay Radio</u>, 306 US 86 ("While*
*a scientific truth, or the mathematical expression of it, is not a*
*patentable invention, a novel and useful structure created with the aid*
*of knowledge of scientific truth may be").*
*The Court in <u>Diehr</u> thus drew a distinction between those claims*
*that "seek to pre-empt the use of" a fundamental principle, on the*
*one hand, and claims that seek only to foreclose others from using*
*a particular "application" of that fundamental principle, on the*
*other. Patents, by definition, grant the power to exclude others from*
*practicing that which the patent claims. <u>Diehr</u> can be understood to*
*suggest that whether a claim is drawn only to a fundamental principle*
*is essentially an inquiry into the scope of that exclusion; i.e., whether*
*the effect of allowing the claim would be to allow the patentee to pre-*
*empt substantially all uses of that fundamental principle. If so, the*
*claim is not drawn to patent-eligible subject matter.*
*In <u>Diehr</u>, the Court held that the claims at issue did not pre-empt all*
*uses of the Arrhenius equation but rather claimed only "a process for*
*curing rubber . . . which incorporates in it a more efficient solution*
*of the equation." The process as claimed included several specific*

*steps to control the curing of rubber more precisely: "These include installing rubber in a press, closing the mold, constantly determining the temperature of the mold, constantly recalculating the appropriate cure time through the use of the formula and a digital computer, and automatically opening the press at the proper time." Thus, one would still be able to use the Arrhenius equation in any process not involving curing rubber, and more importantly, even in any process to cure rubber that did not include performing "all of the other steps in their claimed process." See also Tilgham, 102 US 707 (holding patentable a process of breaking down fat molecules into fatty acids and glycerine in water specifically requiring both high heat and high pressure since other processes, known or as yet unknown, using the reaction of water and fat molecules were not claimed).*

*In contrast to Diehr, the earlier Benson case presented the Court with claims drawn to a process of converting data in binary-coded decimal ("BCD") format to pure binary format via an algorithm programmed onto a digital computer. Benson, 409 US at 65. The Court held the claims to be drawn to unpatentable subject matter: It is conceded that one may not patent an idea. But in practical effect that would be the result if the formula for converting BCD numerals to pure binary numerals were patented in this case. The mathematical formula involved here has no substantial practical application except in connection with a digital computer, which means that if the judgment below is affirmed, the patent would wholly pre-empt the mathematical formula and in practical effect would be a patent on the algorithm itself. Because the algorithm had no uses other than those that would be covered by the claims (i.e., any conversion of BCD to pure binary on a digital computer), the claims pre-empted all uses of the algorithm and thus they were effectively drawn to the algorithm itself. See also O'Reilly, 56 US 62 (holding ineligible a claim pre-empting all uses of electromagnetism to print characters at a distance).*

*The question before us then is whether Applicants' claim recites a fundamental principle and, if so, whether it would pre-empt substantially all uses of that fundamental principle if allowed. Unfortunately, this inquiry is hardly straightforward. How does one determine whether a given claim would pre-empt all uses of a fundamental principle? Analogizing to the facts of Diehr or Benson is of limited usefulness because the more challenging process claims of the twenty-first century are seldom so clearly limited in scope as the highly specific, plainly corporeal industrial manufacturing process of Diehr; nor are they typically as broadly claimed or purely abstract and mathematical as the algorithm of Benson.*

*The Supreme Court, however, has enunciated a definitive test to determine whether a process claim is tailored narrowly enough to encompass only a particular application of a fundamental principle rather than to pre-empt the principle itself. A claimed process is surely patent-eligible under @ 101 if: (1) it is tied to a particular machine or apparatus, or (2) it transforms a particular article into a different state or thing. See <u>Benson</u>, 409 US at 70 ("Transformation and reduction of an article 'to a different state or thing' is the clue to the patentability of a process claim that does not include particular machines."); <u>Diehr</u>, 450 US at 192 (holding that use of mathematical formula in process "transforming or reducing an article to a different state or thing" constitutes patent-eligible subject matter); see also <u>Flook</u>, 437 US at 589 n.9 ("An argument can be made [that the Supreme] Court has only recognized a process as within the statutory definition when it either was tied to a particular apparatus or operated to change materials to a 'different state or thing'"); <u>Cochrane</u>, 94 US 780 ("A process is . . . an act, or a series of acts, performed upon the subject-matter to be transformed and reduced to a different state or thing."). A claimed process involving a fundamental principle that uses a particular machine or apparatus would not pre-empt uses of the principle that do not also use the specified machine or apparatus in the manner claimed. And a claimed process that transforms a particular article to a specified different state or thing by applying a fundamental principle would not pre-empt the use of the principle to transform any other article, to transform the same article but in a manner not covered by the claim, or to do anything other than transform the specified article.*

*The process claimed in <u>Diehr</u>, for example, clearly met both criteria. The process operated on a computerized rubber curing apparatus and transformed raw, uncured rubber into molded, cured rubber products. <u>Diehr</u>, 450 US at 184. The claim at issue in <u>Flook</u>, in contrast, was directed to using a particular mathematical formula to calculate an "alarm limit"—a value that would indicate an abnormal condition during an unspecified chemical reaction. 437 US at 586.*

*The Court rejected the claim as drawn to the formula itself because the claim did not include any limitations specifying "how to select the appropriate margin of safety, the weighting factor, or any of the other variables . . . the chemical processes at work, the [mechanism for] monitoring of process variables, or the means of setting off an alarm or adjusting an alarm system". The claim thus was not limited to any particular chemical (or other) transformation; nor was it tied to any specific machine or apparatus for any of its process steps, such as the selection or monitoring of process variables, or the means of setting off an alarm or adjusting an alarm system". The claim thus was not limited to any particular chemical (or other) transformation; nor was it tied to any specific machine or apparatus for any of its process steps, such as the selection or monitoring of variables or the setting off or adjusting of the alarm.*

*The machine-or-transformation test is a two-branched inquiry; an applicant may show that a process claim satisfies @ 101 either by showing that his claim is tied to a particular machine, or by showing that his claim transforms an article. <u>Benson</u>, 409 US at 70. Certain considerations are applicable to analysis under either branch. First, as illustrated by <u>Benson</u> and discussed below, the use of a specific machine or transformation of an article must impose meaningful limits on the claim's scope to impart patent-eligibility. Second, the involvement of the machine or transformation in the claimed process must not merely be insignificant extra-solution activity. <u>Flook</u>, 437 US at 590. A claimed process is patent-eligible if it transforms an article into a different state or thing. This transformation must be central to the purpose of the claimed process. But the main aspect of the transformation test that requires clarification here is what sorts of things constitute "articles" such that their transformation is sufficient to impart patent-eligibility under @ 101. It is virtually self-evident that a process for a chemical or physical transformation of physical objects or substances is patent-eligible subject matter. As the Supreme Court stated in Benson: [T]he arts of tanning, dyeing, making waterproof cloth, vulcanizing India rubber, smelting ores . . . are instances, however, where the use of chemical substances or physical acts, such as temperature control, changes articles or materials. The chemical process or the physical acts which transform the raw material are, however, sufficiently definite to confine the* *patent monopoly within rather definite bounds. Benson, 409 US at 70. Diehr, 450 US at 184 (process of curing rubber); Tilghman, 102 US at 729 (process of reducing fats into constituent acids and glycerine)".*

(On Bilski's claim)- *"Because the applicable test to determine whether a claim is drawn to a patent-eligible process under @ 101 is the machine-or-transformation test set forth by the Supreme Court and (as) clarified herein, and Applicants' claim here plainly fails that test... the operative question before this court is whether Applicants' claim 1 satisfies the transformation branch of the machine-or-transformation test.*
*We hold that the Applicants' process as claimed does not transform any article to a different state or thing. Purported transformations or manipulations simply of public or private legal obligations or relationships, business risks, or other such abstractions cannot meet the test because they are not physical objects or substances, and they are not representative of physical objects or substances. Applicants' process at most incorporates only such ineligible transformations. See Appellants' Br. at 11 ("[The claimed process] transforms the relationships between the commodity provider, the consumers and market participants ")..., the process as claimed encompasses the exchange of only options, which are simply legal rights to purchase some commodity at a given price in a given time period. The claim only refers to "transactions" involving the exchange of these legal rights at a "fixed rate corresponding to a risk position." Thus, claim 1 does not involve the transformation of any physical object or substance, or an electronic signal representative of any physical object or substance. Given its admitted failure to meet the machine implementation part of the test as well, the claim entirely fails the machine-or-transformation test and is not drawn to patent-eligible subject matter.*
*Applicants' claim is similar to the claims we held unpatentable under @ 101 in Comiskey. There, the applicant claimed a process for mandatory arbitration of disputes regarding unilateral documents and bilateral "contractual" documents in which arbitration was required by the language of the document, a dispute regarding the document was arbitrated, and a binding decision resulted from the arbitration. Comiskey, 499 F.3d at 1368-9. We held the broadest process claims*

*unpatentable under @ 101 because "these claims do not require a machine, and these claims evidently do not describe a process of manufacture or a process for the alteration of a composition of matter.". We concluded that the claims were instead drawn to the "mental process" of arbitrating disputes, and that claims to such an "application of [only] human intelligence to the solution of practical problems" is no more than a claim to a fundamental principle (quoting Benson, 409 US at 67 "[M]ental processes, and abstract intellectual concepts are not patentable, as they are the basic tools of scientific and technological work").*

*Just as the Comiskey claims as a whole were directed to the mental process of arbitrating a dispute to decide its resolution, the claimed process here as a whole is directed to the mental and mathematical process of identifying transactions that would hedge risk. The fact that the claim requires the identified transactions actually to be made does no more to alter the character of the claim as a whole than the fact that the claims in Comiskey required a decision to actually be rendered in the arbitration–i.e., in neither case do the claims require the use of any particular machine or achieve any eligible transformation.*

*We have in fact consistently rejected claims like those in the present appeal and in Comiskey. For example, in Meyer, the applicant sought to patent a method of diagnosing the location of a malfunction in an unspecified multi-component system that assigned a numerical value, a "factor," to each component and updated that value based on diagnostic tests of each component. 688 F.2d at 792-3. The locations of any malfunctions could thus be deduced from reviewing these "factors." The diagnostic tests were not identified, and the "factors" were not tied to any particular measurement; indeed they could be arbitrary. We held that the claim was effectively drawn only to "a mathematical algorithm representing a mental process," and we affirmed the PTO's rejection on @ 101 grounds. No machine was recited in the claim, and the only potential "transformation" was of the disembodied "factors" from one number to another. Thus, the claim effectively sought to pre-empt the fundamental mental process of diagnosing the location of a malfunction in a system by noticing that the condition of a particular component had changed..., a similar claim was rejected in Grams. See 888 F.2d at 839-40 (rejecting claim to process of diagnosing "abnormal condition" in person by identifying and noticing discrepancies in results of unspecified clinical tests of different parts of body).*

*Similarly to the situations in <u>Meyers</u> and <u>Grams</u>, Applicants here seek to claim a non-transformative process that encompasses a purely mental process of performing requisite mathematical calculations without the aid of a computer or any other device, mentally identifying those transactions that the calculations have revealed would hedge each other's risks, and performing the post-solution step of consummating those transactions. Therefore, claim 1 would effectively pre-empt any application of the fundamental concept of hedging and mathematical calculations inherent in hedging (not even limited to any particular mathematical formula). And while Applicants argue that the scope of this pre-emption is limited to hedging as applied in the area of consumable commodities, the Supreme Court's reasoning has made clear that effective pre-emption of all applications of hedging even just within the area of consumable commodities is impermissible. See <u>Diehr</u>, 450 US at 191-2 (holding that field-of-use limitations are insufficient to impart patent-eligibility to otherwise unpatentable claims drawn to fundamental principles). Moreover, while the claimed process contains physical steps (initiating, identifying), it does not involve transforming an article into a different state or thing. Therefore, Applicants' claim is not drawn to patent-eligible subject matter under @ 101".*

ii. "..plaintiff has not yet received 'final agency action' sufficient to provide the court with jurisdiction under the APA. Moreover, Congress has clearly channeled all Article III judicial review of USPTO patent rejections into.. Fed Cir. and USDC/DC" (p.2-4).

<u>Response</u>: Whether or not USPTO issued a final rejection on my pending Patent-application has <u>no</u> relevance to the jurisdiction of this court under APA. See Supreme Court ruling in <u>Norton</u>, 542 US 55, cite at 2 iii above. If the defendant's intent, here, is to persuade this court to dismiss my claim under APA by *twisting* or *misusing* the facts-law, and possibly prolong resolution of this matter, it is <u>not</u> fair in the interest of the Public whose interests must be paramount to the defendant, the court, and to all of us..

iii. "..in August 2009, the USPTO issued a document entitled Interim Examination Instructions for Evaluating Subject Matter Eligibility Under 35 USC 101. In the very first paragraph of the document, the USPTO articulated both the rationale that animated the dissemination of the Interim Guidance, and the non-binding nature of the same…" (p.6).

Response: *First*, why issue an 'Interim Guidance' at Public expense, if it is a non-binding document 'upon *substantive law*', the *examiner* or the *patentee*. However, the Relevant-*facts* at 1 i-iii & 1 xi-xiii, show USPTO did use this Interim Guidance selectively to deprive my rights; and, it failed to correct the wrongful-acts despite my timely objection or response. That shows Fed Cir. judges' words are on point in Tafas, 559 F.3d 1345 (2009)-

*"While the text of the rules sets forth a facially reasonable procedural requirement, we are mindful of the possibility that the USPTO may in some cases attempt to apply the rules in a way that makes compliance essentially impossible and substantively deprives applicants of their rights. In such cases, judicial review will be available under 5 USC @ 706"*.

*Second*, everything in our-Universe, seen and unseen, is in a constant *flux*; so, USPTO to consider the subject matter eligibility is in flux should not be a surprise, although that is not true under Biliski. Otherwise after Biliski come Prometheus and another… while the Public suffering (sleeplessly or with drugs…) night after night and year after year continues.

iv. "A new examiner reviewed the application, and on June 20, 2008, issued an office action initially rejecting plaintiff's proposed patent claims on the same grounds… And once again, a new examiner reviewed the application, and in October 2009 issued the same initial rejections.." (p.8).

Response: The so called new examiner twice-mentioned is the same, Mr.Gilbert, electrical engineer, who did reject my Patent claims twice per the dictates of *in-house authority*; and, he took that position second time using this so called non-binding Interim Guidance… Should the USPTO deny this fact, a quick discovery must proceed.

v. ".. plaintiff's claim in this court is somewhat unclear. On this score, plaintiff's complaint provides that the USPTO 'discriminated' against him and his 'Method' when it suddenly came up with a new rule in August 2009, without giving me, a person with application in cold storage, an opportunity to participate in this new rulemaking, and knowingly incorporated one-sentence in the new rules to stop me from getting Patent, and give a free hand to drug-makers..." (p.9).

Response: The Relevant-*facts* I stated and the Relevant-*law* I cited show USPTO's discrimination against me and my method at every-step on the way for nearly 4-years. It came-up with this one-sentence substantive-change in the rule and made it effective on August 24, 2009 while keeping my Patent-application in a cold-storage for nearly a year (Exhibit 3.6), then applied that rule in a way to make my compliance essentially impossible, and deprived my rights. Furthermore, such discrimination of giving a free hand to the drug-makers can be seen in Prometheus, 581 F.3d 1336, where a Patent is granted for a 'method or *process*' in the absence of showing data whether it met the 'machine or *transformation*' test (see Exhibit 5 on p.6/6). Discovery will provide evidence on such discrimination...

vi. "Plaintiff therefore could have submitted comments on the Interim Guidance both before and after the examiner issued his initial, non-final rejections... the USPTO provided an opportunity to comment in any event, plaintiff has failed to state a claim upon which relief can be granted.." (p.15).

Response: As stated I did submit my comments on time (although I am not aware of USPTO's Notice at that time...); but, USPTO failed to act or repeal the substantive change in the rule it made effective on August 24, 2009. Therefore, a claim is stated upon which relief can be granted by this court.

vii. "The USPTO also provided that any and all claim 'rejections are and will continue to be based upon the substantive law, and it is those rejections that are appealable'... the agency explicitly recognized in this very context, it is the binding precedent from its supervisory courts that governs the ultimate question of patentability, not the

Interim Guidance... <u>Animal Legal</u>, which binds this court, requires a finding that Interim Guidance is an 'interpretative rule' exempt from the APA's notice and comment requirements" (p.14).

<u>Response</u>: That's fine.., but the record here makes it clear examiner Gilbert did issue a non-final rejection in my case on the basis of the substantive law made in USPTO's Interim Guidance; and USPTO failed to repeal the new-rule or correct Mr.Gilbert's use or misuse upon my objections. In <u>Tafas</u>, 559 F.3d 1345 (2009), Fed. Cir. (*en banc*) analyzed the distinction between '*substantive*', procedural or '*interpretive*' rule-making by USPTO and said (in judges' own words)-
"*We agree.. that @2(b)(2) does not vest the USPTO with any general substantive rulemaking power. This principle is amply supported by our precedent, <u>Animal Legal</u>, 932 F.2d 920 (A substantive declaration with regard to the Commissioner's interpretation of the patent statutes, whether it be sec. 101, 102, 103, 112 or other section, does not fall within the usual interpretation of [the language in <u>sec. 6</u>, the predecessor of <u>@2(b)(2)]); <u>Cooper Techs.</u>, 536 F.3d 1330 (To comply with <u>sec. 2(b)(2)(A)</u>, a Patent Office rule must be 'procedural'–i.e., it must 'govern the conduct of proceedings in the Office)... Accordingly, we must **reject** the USPTO's argument that the substantive/procedural distinction is immaterial in this case.*
*Substantive rules certainly "affect individual rights and obligations," but that inquiry does not necessarily distinguish most procedural requirements, which will also "affect individual rights and obligations." The Supreme Court itself made this observation when drawing the line between "substance" and "procedure" in the context of the Rules Enabling Act, <u>Hanna</u>, 380 US 460 (Undoubtedly most alterations of the rules of practice and procedure may and often do affect the rights of litigants)... While this court has previously evaluated USPTO rules in terms of whether they "affect individual rights and obligations," it has done so in the process of distinguishing between "interpretive" and "substantive" rules, <u>Animal Legal</u>, 932 F.2d 927; <u>Cooper</u>, 536 F.3d 1336. We agree, ... that while the inquiry set forth in <u>Chrysler</u> and used in <u>Animal</u> and <u>Cooper</u> may be useful in defining the boundary between interpretive and substantive rules, it is not dispositive on the issue of whether the final rules are procedural...*

*We are most persuaded in this case by the D.C. Circuit's approach in JEM, 22 F.3d 326-328. At issue in that case were "hard look" rules adopted by the Federal Communications Commission ("FCC") in response to a significant number of "carelessly prepared and speculative applications" for broadcasting licenses. Under those rules, applications that either failed to include necessary information or contained incorrect or inconsistent information that could not be "resolved within the confines of the application and with a high degree of confidence" were dismissed with no opportunity to cure the defect. The D.C. Circuit rejected JEM's contention that the rules were substantive because they "deprive[d] license applicants of the opportunity to correct errors or defects in their filings." In doing so, the court noted that a "critical feature of the procedural exception [in sec. 553 of the APA] is that it covers agency actions that do not themselves alter the rights or interests of parties, although [they] may alter the manner in which the parties present themselves or their viewpoints to the agency."... The "critical fact" that was "fatal to JEM's claim," the court held, was that the "hard look" rules "did not change the substantive standards by which the FCC evaluates license applications." The court recognized that the rules could result in the loss of substantive rights, but found that they were nonetheless procedural because they did not "foreclose effective opportunity to make one's case on the merits."*

*While we do not purport to set forth a definitive rule for distinguishing between substance and procedure in this case, we conclude that the final rules challenged in this case are procedural. In essence, they govern the timing of and materials that must be submitted with patent applications. The final rules may "alter the manner in which the parties present . . . their viewpoints" to the USPTO, but they do not, on their face, "foreclose effective opportunity" to present patent applications for examination... While the text of the rules sets forth a facially reasonable procedural requirement, we are mindful of the possibility that the USPTO may in some cases attempt to apply the rules in a way that makes compliance essentially impossible and substantively deprives applicants of their rights. In such cases, judicial review will be available under 5 USC @ 706".*

*Conclusion*:

The facts, the law and my argument above stated a claim upon which this court can grant relief, and this court has jurisdiction in the matter under APA.

I request the court (1) help settle the matter expeditiously in the interest of the Public; or (2A) enter an order under 5 USC @ 706(2) to hold unlawful and set aside USPTO's substantive rule in 'Interim Guidance' as arbitrary, capricious, an abuse of discretion, contrary to constitutional right, power, privilege; and in excess of statutory jurisdiction, authority; and (2B) enter a declaratory-order under 28 USC @ 2201(a) that the one-sentence new-rule in the 'Interim Guidance' is being *applied against this applicant in a way that makes his compliance essentially impossible and substantively deprives his right*, therefore, in the interest of Public, expedite review of his pending Patent-application by an examiner with expertise in transformation of brain-neurons or Mr.Pezzuto with bio-medical expertise who is positive in 2007 (until the in-house authority dictates…).

Respectfully,

I, M.R. Mikkilineni, the applicant in the Patent-application No.12/259,285 and a person whose rights are deprived under USPTO's substantive rulemaking on August 24, 2009, swear to state that the alleged relevant-facts in this pleading (and in my complaint) and the documents attached are true and correct to the best of my knowledge, information and belief.

M.R.Mikkilineni
PO Box 32110, Washington, DC 20007

I certify that I hand delivered a copy of this pleading on April 15, 2010 to the office of US attorney ED of Va. at-
Mr.DC Barghaan, Esq. Assist. US attorney
2100 Jamieson Ave. Alexandria, Va. 22314

**UNITED STATES DISTRICT COURT** FOR *EASTREN DISTRICT OF VARGINIA*

M.R.Mikkilineni
      Plaintiff,
v.

                    No:09cv1412
                    Judge Brinkema

Robert Stoll, Commissioner for Patents
      Defendant.

**Plaintiff's *Reply* to Defendants' *Memorandum of law* of 04/21/2010**

Dear Honorable Judge:
I did not, yet, receive in the US mail a copy of defendants' pleading filed on April 21, 2010, although Mr.Barghaan was kind to e-mail me a copy on Friday, 04/23/2010 at 3pm at my request.

Like President Reagan used to say *"here, we go again"*, defendant again took the same '*old*' twisted path mostly with irrelevant arguments that-

"Congress through the patent act has provided an elaborate remedial system...plaintiff here, first to wait (for) a final rejection of (patent) from a USPTO examiner, then proceed with an appeal to the Board... and only then obtain...judicial review (in Fed Cir. or USDC/DC)... this court lacks jurisdiction"
It went on and on... informing that *only* the defendant knows what is *right* or *wrong* and this court should stay out of this issue because 5 USC @ 553 is a '*dead letter*' with no teeth to bite. See Commonwealth v. US, 2009 US Dist. LEXIS 110293 (2009, USDC/DC) citing Sugar Cane Growers, 289 F.3d 89 (DC Cir.).

However, defendant did not or could not dispute any of the facts or law I cited, including on the key-issue at hand-Whether USPTO has '*failed to take a discrete action*', which it is required to take upon receiving my timely comments, to repeal a '*substantive*' rule or change in policy made effective on August 24, 2009, before notice and public comment; the policy it used against me for nearly 4-years, *first* through the '*in-house authority*' in the absence of a formal change in the rule, and *now* with an official-change in the policy which made my compliance essentially impossible and substantively deprived my rights. See 5 USC @ 553(c), (d) & (e), and 706(2); Norton, 542 US 55; Tafas, 559 F.3d 1345 (2009, Fed. Cir.)

Instead, defendant is attempting to side track the key-issue at hand and said- F*irst* (p.2) "USPTO responding to the only claim that plaintiff actually presented (that USPTO failed to provide notice and allow for public comment)"; and *second* (p.3-4) "plaintiff… seeking to have this court set aside a single sentence in the Interim Guidance on its merits… plaintiff now asks this court to wade into the uncertain waters of substantive patent law… Nothing within plaintiff's complaint.. proffered such a challenge"

See under jurisdiction- in my complaint I cited:
(1) @ 553(c) 'agency shall give interested persons an opportunity to participate in the rule making…', on which defendant admits to *not* given that opportunity to me before the effective date of August 24, 2009, at least on that *one single-sentence* of *substantive-rule* in its Interim Guidance that directly affects my rights; and
(2) @ 553(e) 'agency shall give an interested person the right to petition for the issuance, amendment, or repeal of a rule', on which the record shows defendant has *failed* to act or did not issue, amend, or repeal that *one sentence* of *substantive-rule* that is being used against me to make my compliance essentially impossible and substantively depriving my rights. Also, with the cite-
(3) @ 706(2) to 'hold agency action unlawful and set aside findings and conclusions…', (see complaint, under conclusion) I requested the court for an *order to invalidate or strike that one-sentence in the new-rule which is placed solely to stop me from giving people an inexpensive, good and healthy choice..'*
The facts alleged in my complaint and subsequently clarified in my memorandum of law are written in simple English (not in *Sanskrit*, our-*root* language…). So, there is no reason for this defendant to call my claim a *new* APA challenge…or claim I am asking the court to "wade into the uncertain waters…", unless defendant wanted a

second bite of the apple to create more confusion as it did, and thus make the day.

It is not surprising defendant wants this court to *forget* Tafas, 559 F.3d 1345 (2009, Fed. Cir. *en banc*) because-
(1) USPTO had to *rescind* the rules that formed the basis of that litigation (both *substantive* and *procedural* new-rules); and

(2) That court said- "While the text of the rules sets forth a facially reasonable procedural requirement, we are mindful of the possibility that the USPTO may in some cases attempt to apply the rules in a way that makes compliance essentially impossible and substantively deprives applicants of their rights. In such cases, judicial review will be available under 5 USC @ 706".
And, defendant wants this court to *adopt* as the binding-rule, an older-case Animal, 932 F.2d 920 (1991, Fed. Cir.)-
(1) Where the court dismissed that appeal for 'lack of standing'; and
(2) That court said (at 927)- "A rule is substantive when it effects a change in existing law or policy which affect[s] individual rights and obligations... In contrast, a rule which merely clarifies or explains existing law or regulations is interpretative".
Even if this court adopts Animal as binding, the record in my case makes it clear USPTO used a discriminatory policy against me for nearly 4-years, *first* through the '*in-house authority*' in the absence of a formal change in the rule, and *now* with an official or formal change in the policy, which makes my compliance essentially impossible and substantively deprives my rights.
It is beyond comprehension how this defendant can keep claiming, with a straight-face:
(1) The *one sentence* new-*rule* or policy that "*purely mental processes in which thoughts or human based actions are 'changed' are not considered an eligible transformation*" is not substantive, but interpretative only because defendant said that-(it) "...
simply intending to clarify the confusion that might exist in the various existing judicial interpretations of @ 101's limits on patentable subject matter" (p.7); although it did not explain what is that confusion and how this one sentence clarified... And, the defendant knew-

(2)  <u>No</u> court in the land has <u>ever</u> made a ruling similar to that one sentence rule which USPTO's own *in-house authority* simply made it up…as if defendant can take '*any position under the Sun…*', and the affected person or this court should accept that position because defendant stated that it is "*fully consistent with biding precedent*"; or-
(3)  Defendant "*stated that it was not engaging in substantive rulemaking*".
In <u>Prometheus,</u> 581 F.3d 1336 (2009, Fed. Cir.) *re*-affirmed that under 35 USC @ 101 *Congress intended statutory subject matter to include anything under the Sun* [see complaint at 9(iii)]; so, Congress did not authorize USPTO to take '*any position under the Sun*' in making a new-policy and reject patent selectively at will, like in my case.

Once more defendant goes back to <u>Animal</u> and claims "*sec. 101… does not turn on any discretion residing in examiners*" (p.8). I do not dispute that in my case. In fact, the facts in the record make it clear- that to be the truth- *first* the *in-house* authority and *then* USPTO has dictated the out come, and the examiner simply followed those dictates without using any discretion or expertise of his-own. Defendant did not rest there; it decided to switch gears and try a different route to defend its own wrongful-acts of nearly 4-years. It does not matter who gets injured in its path, and wants me to go on with the appeals (for another 5 or more years and said-
"the interim guidance regarding the interpretation of @ 101 is no way binding on either the Fed. Cir. or USDC/DC (or the Board)… as such, even were USPTO examiners bound by the interim guidance, because the courts are not so bound, plaintiff's purported rights to patent his sleep method are not ultimately impacted by the interim guidance" Elegantly said, but makes no-sense in reality; if this defendant can *go free* with such arguments there is no end… and this could become a habit. USPTO can simply create interim guidance with a new-policy and take any '*position under the sun*' claiming 'flux', whenever its *in-house authority* decides '*not to grant patent*' to any others out of "*thousands* of other patent applicants". That would cause havoc to Article III courts… if jurisdiction under @ 553 & 706 is surrendered as defendant wants in my case. As an example in real-life: a street thug or drug-addict attempts to snatch purse from a helpless girl at gun-point, and he notices an officer's car coming his way; the guy

stops his act and convinces the officer 'to *go away* because *nothing is happening...*, if something... happens, *she can report to an officer...*' (the girl scared and agrees...). The officer walks away... and the guy finishes his act... the result would not be pretty... Such incidents multiply in no time to cause havoc on the judicial system. Likewise, here, the defendant is persuading this curt to walk away from @ 553 & 706, and inviting me to commit for a continued injury at the expense of Public-interest...

I requested this court primarily to review defendants' *failure to act* under @ 553(c), (e) and @ 706(2), not on 'agency's patentability decisions' or to 'review the examiner's non-final rejection' that belong to Article III courts (p.9-11). I did not 'elect' to change "focus" of inquiry to eliminate Congress' intent; because the interim guidance contains a substantive-rule or new-policy which affects my rights and obligations, this court has jurisdiction to go into the merits to the extent necessary for a finding on the issue of defendants' continued discrimination against me using that one-sentence substantive change in policy.

When discovery discloses new-evidence on USPTO's nearly one-year delay to issue a non-final rejection, or the continued delay since December 2009 with regard to the final-action on my application, I will amend my complaint, if required, to include a claim under @ 706(1) for "unreasonably delaying" and/or for other claims.

Upon my inquiry, I am informed (on phone) by an employee of the Board that 'the Board is part of USPTO, as such it has no-power to strike any new-rule or change in policy... even if that change affected rights of applicants'. Therefore, defendants' cite (p.12) that "the Board is not bound by such guidelines" is a matter open for discovery.

Finally, I have not asked this court to ignore Congress' clear mandate with regard to the patent Act; and, there is no law that authorizes this court to walk away and make Congress' law @ 553, a "*dead letter*". Defendant is the one persuading this court to ignore Congress' clear mandate under APA.... One should wonder- why this dependent wants to prolong the agony when there is a simple solution to the issue- agree to repeal the discriminatory policy- move on in the interest of Public...

In *conclusion*, I request this Honorable court to deny defendants' motion to dismiss because this court has jurisdiction and my claim under APA is real. I request the court to make sense to the defendant, and help settle this matter in the interest of Public- at 71, I have no other interest. Or enter an order to set aside or strike that one-sentence new-rule...; or allow discovery.

Respectfully,

M.R.Mikkilineni
PO Box 32110
Washington, DC 20007

I certify that I hand delivered a copy of this pleading on April 25, 2010 to the office of US attorney ED of Va. at- US attorney, 2100 Jamieson Ave., Alexandria, Va. 22314

**UNITED STATES DISTRICT COURT** FOR *EASTREN DISTRICT OF VARGINIA*

M.R.Mikkilineni
      Plaintiff,

v.

                                     No:09cv1412
                                     Judge Brinkema

Robert Stoll, Commissioner for Patents
      Defendant.

**Plaintiff's *Motion* for *Re-hearing* on the *merits* and to *amend* or *void* Order of April 30, 2010**

Dear judge Brinkema:
On April 30, 2010, I spoke to a clerk in your office- she is nice to tell me-
'*You can file a motion to amend the Order within 28-days from the date of the Order, and you can also appeal within 60-days*'. I assume those are your directions because she put me on hold for few-minutes before telling me that.
So, I hereby file this motion for re-hearing, and a Notice of Appeal to the Fed. Cir. on this May 17, 2010- I will give a telephone call to your office to find if you are willing to consider this request- if so, I will give a notice to US attorney regarding the hearing date- if not, let the appeal proceed.
In support of my request I state as follows:

*Evidence*:  (from court-reporter's transcript filed...)
1.  You asked US attorney- "Is there any additional argument... you want to put on the record?" He said- "*No, your Honor*" (p.2, L24).
As if *false*-argument alone matters, *not* the relevant-evidence in the record...; and, you did not give the same opportunity to me or let me present evidence either.

2.  Then, you and he talked about "*final rejection*" and my "*ability to appeal*" (p.3, L24)-

The record shows *final rejection* of patent or my *ability to appeal* is irrelevant to the issue before you to decide under 5 USC @ 553 & 706(2); but, your line of inquiry is clearly intended to make the relevant statute a '*dead letter*' and thrash a recent-ruling in Commonwealth v. US, 2009 US Dist. LEXIS 110293 (2009, USDC/ DC, citing Sugar Cane Growers, 289 F.3d 89 (DC Cir.))- this is *not* interpreting a statute, but it is making a *new*-law from the bench while thrashing Congress and the Americans:

(i) You said- "by filing this complaint, under the Patent Office's practice, stopped.. evaluation…" His response- "*when an Article III case is filed regarding a particular patent application, …they will stop prosecution… That is not a hard-and-fast rule …they have applied that rule in this context..*" (p.4, L1-12).
You and he knew, being lawyers, PTO has absolutely *no*-authority under the statute to make-up "that *rule*"……
(ii) You said- ".. the interpretive guidance (PTO) issued while they await the Supreme Court to resolve or… address Fed. Cir.'s latest ruling on method…" His response- "*PTO made very clear that because it is an interpretive rule, it's not substantive rule making…*" (p.4, L15-24).
The evidence I presented, which is in the court-record, makes absolutely clear that under the guise of interpretive rules PTO included at least '*one substantive-rule*' and deprived my rights…

(iii) At that point you made a conclusion- "the way law is set up, this court and no Article III court has the ability to rewrite the interpretive rules" of PTO.
His answer- "*That's correct*" (p.5, L7-10).
My pending-claim in this case under 5 USC @706(2) is not "*to rewrite the interpretive rules*", but "*to set aside that one substantive rule*", that PTO has used or misused against me (for 4-years), deprived me of my rights, and thus negligently caused injury to about 35% of the Americans that suffer with insomnia or the drugs, and even face-*death* like Michael Jackson….

(iv) Then you raised the issue of "proper procedure… due process issue… failure to provide notice…". He agreed- "*the Fed. Cir... has the authority to tell PTO that its interpretive guidance is wrong"* (p.5, L12-3 & L19-21).

You said- "On the merits". He agreed- *"correct"* (p.5, L22-3).

Although this court or an Article III court has the ability under 5 USC @706(2) *to set aside a substantive rule...*, you did *not* go into the *merits*. You sought the job of a judge, and agreed to *serve* Americans in the name of Almighty-god; so, you have a *duty* to get to the 'merits' in this case before you make conclusions.....

(v) But, you concluded- "It's not an abstract process where there's been no final rejection..." (p.6, L22-3). He said- *"there would be no standing for an individual...unless there was some reasonable expectation that it would be applied against them in a detrimental way..."* (p.7, L1-3).
I made that absolutely clear in my briefs that the issue of *'final rejection'* is a *non-issue* under 5 USC @553 & 706(2), because my claim is based on PTO's *use or misuse of a substantive rule against me in a detrimental way...*

3. Then, you said to me- "the reality of it is that the lawsuit that you have filed in this court and the motion..., have no legal foundation. As the gov. has correctly pointed out, you have not yet had a final agency action... patent has not finally been rejected... by filing this lawsuit, basically you stopped that process... without a final action from the agency, you really have no basis to be in this court (p.7, L12-24)... All we would be concerned... is whether the process was appropriate... under concepts of due process,..., there's absolutely nothing in your case to indicate that there's been anything amiss in how the matters have been handled (p.8, L16-21).... For these reasons defendant's motion to dismiss is granted. This case is dismissed. Your motion to set aside the substantive rule is denied (p.9, L6-8).

4. Transcript shows- you did *not* allow me to *speak*, or *respond* to any of those irrelevant-issues you and US attorney talked about; you did *not* allow me to *present* my motion to *set aside* the *substantive rule...*

You did *not* allow *discovery* in the matter despite my request in the pleadings. You did *not* allow a *hearing* on my evidence or the arguments I presented in my pleadings...

You made up your mind simply based on *false*-arguments PTO made on lack of '*final rejection*' and my *ability* to appeal. That's it....

5. Then, your Order of 30$^{th}$ April 2010 (which I received on 05/04/2010) said- "defendant's motion to dismiss is granted and plaintiff's motion to set aside PTO's substantive rule & declaratory order is denied... this civil action is dismissed with prejudice..."

**In doing so, you did <u>not</u> even consider to help <u>settle</u> the issue amicably despite my request...**

<u>*Argument*</u>:

Defendant did *not* ask my case be "*dismissed with prejudice*". In fact, your own proclamation in the court said- "*This case is dismissed*" (p.9, L7).

But, your Order appears to be made with '*bias and prejudice*', *first* against me, and *second* against the 35% of Americans- with an outright *denial* of a hearing on the *merits* in the case. Thus, not *only* PTO denied due process, but you too *did* the same by accepting PTO's *false*-arguments....

In the process you bypassed the key-issue I raised to decide- "Whether USPTO has '*failed to take a discrete action*', which it is required to take upon receiving my timely comments, to repeal a '*substantive*' rule or change in policy made effective on August 24, 2009, before notice and public comment- the policy it used against me for nearly 4-years, *first* through the '*in-house authority*' in the absence of a formal change in the rule, and *now* with an official-change in the policy which made my compliance essentially impossible and substantively deprived my rights under 5 USC @ 553(c), (d) & (e), and 706(2)". See <u>Norton</u>, 542 US 55; <u>Tafas</u>, 559 F.3d 1345 (2009, Fed. Cir.).

Therefore, I request a *re*-hearing 'on the *merits*'; and allow me to present evidence directly relevant to the key-issue in the case, in the interest of judicial economy and prompt resolution of the matter...

Respectfully,

M.R.Mikkilineni
PO Box 32110
Washington, DC 20007

I certify that I hand delivered a copy of this pleading on May 17, 2010 to the office of US attorney ED of Va. at- US attorney, 2100 Jamieson Ave., Alexandria, Va. 22314

**UNITED STATES COURT OF APPEALS** FOR THE FEDERAL
Cir.

**No. 2010-1362**

M.R.Mikkilineni
        Plaintiff-Appellant,
v.

Robert STOLL, Commissioner of Patents,
        Defendant-Appellee.

Appeal from the United States District Court for the Eastern District
of Virginia, Case No. 09-cv-1412, Judge Leonie M. Brinkema.

*Informal Brief of Appellant* (Appendix attached)

On June 15, 2010, I file one original and three copies of *signed* 2-
page informal brief with 20-extra sheets to answer questions 1-6, plus
55- pages of docket entries (DE) & Exhibits for review and a decision
in the matter by this Honorable court.

**1.** *Relevant* Facts:
(i)  Sometime in 2005-6, I perfected an idea how to activate
the '*master clock*' in my brain for a sleep-cycle by flipping off
the '*light-switch*' in the brain-stem, and fall asleep *instantly*.
The '*process*' is a tune-up of the brain to *transform specific-
neurons* into a different state, and make them active in producing
melatonin and serotonin to activate the *master clock* for a sleep-
cycle by flipping off *the light-switch*; and, the '*process*' works
this way-

"*Learn to generate positive-signals* (electrical) *using specific
positive-thoughts in the mind, input those signals into the brain-
algorithm* (brain circuits, like data input into the computer
machine-code ...) *and process those signals in the neurons* (like
processing in the chips...) *to get transformed* and *induce sleep-
cycle*"

The *'process'* tunes the brain off of excited negative-signals generated by natural phenomena of streaming intrusive thoughts into the mind as a result of anxiety, anger, depression or mental-disorder(s).

Brain has two hemispheres and one is dominant; the two hemispheres communicate with each other, one thought at a time. Any interference from two or more thoughts in the mind, at the same instant or time, creates havoc with motor responses in the brain; and the two hemispheres stop communicating- a split brain. That split brain causes the *light switch* 'flip' in the brain-stem to activate the *master-clock* and make brain fall-asleep; and helps cure depression or mental-disorder(s).

(ii) Brain is the control center of the body; it controls thought-signals, senses, memory and function of cells and organs. Survival depends on a properly functioning brain to regulate the functions of the organs; and it requires a sleep-cycle of about 8-hours in a 24-hour day to function properly. A recent study at Harvard Medical School and University of California concludes-

*"...a lack of sleep causes the brain's emotional centers to dramatically overreact...(with) psychiatric disorders... (and) fractures the brain mechanisms that regulate key aspects of mental health... and, sleep appears to restore emotional brain's circuits...."*

The National Sleep Foundation's (NSF) sleep in America poll found that 74% of American adults experience sleep problems a few nights a week or more, 39% get less than seven hours of sleep each weeknight, and more than one in three (35%) are so sleepy during the day that it interferes with daily activities. 1 in 10 suffers from chronic insomnia and it is estimated that sleeplessness costs the US economy $35 billion a year....

(iii) The sleep problems arise from changes in the brain regions and neurons that control sleep, or from the drugs used to control other disorders. Currently, there are several drugs available to aid sleep; and possible side effects include feeling tired or drowsy the next day, memory loss, headache and problems with performance. Prescription sleeping pills can cause strange and potentially dangerous side effects. And, such side effects can include dangerous allergic reactions and bizarre behaviors such as sleep eating, walking and driving, in which a person will drive a car while not fully awake and has no memory of doing so.

(iv)  At this stage, science is trying to find a way to implant a new *'gene'* or *light switch* in the brain for treating mental-disorder(s), and/or to control sleep-wake state of the brain with a flip of the *light switch*; but, science is unable to locate or 'repair' the *light switch* that exists in the brain-stem.  My *'process'* or method is able to 'repair' the *light switch* and make it work <u>without</u> an implant or use of a pill or drug.

**2.** *Undisputed* material-facts:

(i)  On June 08, 2006, **4**- years ago, I made an application for Patent to USPTO (at No.11/449,519); because, if I place my method into practice or start a teaching school, without Patent protection, the pill or drug makers could start a parallel organization and drive me out, and keep making money selling pills or drugs.

(ii)  On December 21, 2006, my petition is granted to make 'special' or expedite review because of my *ill*-health; on Jan. 17, 2007, examiner sent claim rejections (non-final) under 35 USC @101, as *non-statutory subject matter*; under 35 USC @112 paras.1-2, as failing to comply with *enablement requirement* and failing to *define* the invention… Mr.Swift, Esq., a patent-attorney (whom I hired with limited-funds I saved out of my SS) timely responded to the rejections with an amendment.

(iii)  On May 30, 2007, Mr.Swift and I met Mr.Pezzuto, supervisor-Examiner and discussed the issues.  Mr.Pezzuto's interview summary stated *"there is no agreement as the rejection under 35 USC 101 and the examiner will discuss this with in-house authorities"* (Exhibit 1.3).

Later, Mr.Pezzuto indicated likelihood of granting Patent- but, on October 12, 2007, a Jr. Examiner (working for Pezzuto) sent a **final** rejection per the *dictates* of *in-house authority*.

(iv) On December 06, 2007, I filed another application (at No.11/999,349), a 'continuation in part' (CiP1); my application is sent to a new-Examiner. On August 07, 2008, I met examiner Gilbert and explained how one interested in the skill can be trained to use the method for useful result; Mr.Gilbert understood it and his interview summary stated (Exhibit 2.4A)-

*"Mr.Mikkilineni explained that his method was not concentrating on a scene with two elements of an image at the same time, but, keep two separate elements as two separate thoughts,* (and) *bring them into the mind at the same time"*.

I made it clear that a specification or a book can't teach some-one to ride a bike, or an MD-trainee do brain-Surgery on the first-day without proper training…; and if books can enable an ordinary skilled to do it, there is no need for teaching schools.

On June 20, 2008, Examiner sent me claim rejections (non-final) under 35 USC @101, as *non-statutory subject matter*; under 35 USC @112 paras. 1-2, as *failing to comply with enablement requirement and as being indefinite claim…*, as before.

On September 19, 2008, I had a telephone interview with supervisor-Examiner Marmor, and his summary says (Exhibit 2.4)-

*"Applicant explained… and suggested a sleep study be conducted to address the rejections… examiner explained that the sleep study would likely **not be useful**… that the pending method claims involve **merely mental steps** and are unpatentable and **nonstatutory**. A patent eligible process under 35 USC 101 must be tied to another statutory class, such as a particular apparatus, or **transform** underlying subject matter or material"*.

My method is <u>not</u> *"merely mental steps"*- but, USPTO's *in-house authority* mislabeled to *dictate* the out come and *kill* it.

(v) On October 27, 2008, Mr.Swift, Esq., patent-attorney, filed a new application (at No.12/259,285), a 'continuation in part' (CiP2);

and, on March 10, 2009, my petition is granted to make 'special' or expedite review based on age.

On September 21, 2009, I discovered an article published in Washington Post titled '*Meditation Gives Brain a Charge…*'- a study conducted at U. of Wisconsin with the help of **Dalai Lama** (the study-results were published by **National Academy of Sciences**); I forwarded that to examiner Gilbert (Exhibit 3.3).

(vi)  On October 01, 2009, examiner Gilbert sent claim *rejection* (non-final) under 35 USC @101, as *inoperative and lacks utility*; and under 35 USC @112 paras. 1-2, as failing to comply with *enablement requirement* and as being *indefinite* claim etc.., as before (Exhibit 3.4).

Examiner issued this rejection under 35 USC @ 101 (on Oct. 01, 2009) knowing-

**. human brain, a physical object contains neurons- physical substance; and, my method transforms the neurons which stopped working into a different state to enable them work and produce melatonin and serotonin for a sleep cycle; and**

. on September 16, 2009, Fed Cir. (see PROMETHEUS v. MAYO, 581 F.3d 1336) *re-affirmed* that under 35 USC 101 Congress intended statutory subject matter to include anything under the sun that is made by man, and clarified that-

"*a claimed process is surely patent-eligible under @101 if: it transforms a particular article into a different state.. the patentee may show that a process claim satisfies @101 by showing that his claim transforms an article…This transformation must be central to the purpose of the claimed process. It is virtually self-evident that a process for a chemical or physical transformation of physical objects or substances is patent-eligible subject matter… After all, even though a fundamental principle itself is not patent-eligible, processes incorporating a fundamental principle may be patent-eligible" under 35 USC @101…The invention's purpose **to treat the human body is made clear in the specification** and the* *preambles of the asserted claims... the* **human body necessarily undergoes a transformation***... quite* **literally every transformation of physical matter can be described as occurring according to natural processes and natural law. Transformations operate by natural principles.** *The transformation here, however, is the result of the* **physical administration** *of a drug to a subject* **to transform—** *i.e.,* **treat–the subject, which is itself not a natural process.** *It is* **virtually self-evident that a process for a chemical or physical transformation of physical objects or substances is patent-eligible subject matter...** See Diehr at 187 ("Their process admittedly employs a well-known mathematical equation, but they do not seek to preempt the use of that equation; rather, they seek only to foreclose from others the use of that equation in conjunction with all of the other steps in their claimed process."). *Regardless, because the claims meet the machine-or-transformation test, they do not preempt a fundamental principle.* See Bilski at 954 (characterizing the machine-or-transformation test as "a definitive test to determine whether a process is tailored narrowly enough to encompass only a particular application of a fundamental principle rather than to pre-empt the principle itself")".

*"The inventive nature of the claimed methods stems not from preemption of all use of these natural processes, but from the application of a natural phenomenon in a series of transformative steps comprising particular methods of treatment. A claimed process that transforms a particular article to a specified different state or thing by applying a fundamental principle would not pre-empt the use of the principle to transform any other article, to transform the same article but in a manner not covered by the claim, or to do anything other than transform the specified article. It is clear that these methods of treatment are @ 101 patentable subject matter."*

And, examiner Gilbert issued this rejection under 35 USC @ 112 (on Oct. 01, 2009), knowing-

. **my specification conveyed with reasonable clarity to a skilled person in the art, with a degree** (plus experience) **in** '*sleep medicine*', **to understand I am in possession of the claimed**

**invention on the filing date, and the best mode to carry out my invention is the teaching school; and**

. on June 28, 2007, Fed. Cir. said (see <u>Hyatt</u> v. Dudas, 492 F.3d 1365)-

Under 35 USC @ 112 *"adequate written description means that, in the specification, the applicant must convey with reasonable clarity to those skilled in the art that, as of the filing date sought, he or she was **in possession of the claimed invention**... This is not to say that the PTO can reject a complex claim with numerous limitations by summarily declaring that no written description support exists... the examiner to specify which claim limitation is lacking adequate support in the written description"*

. on October 12, 2007, Fed Cir.'s said (see <u>ALLVOICE</u> v. NUANCE, 504 F.3d 1236)-

*"The definiteness requirement is set forth at 35 USC @ 112 para.2: The specification shall conclude with one or more claims particularly pointing out and distinctly claiming the subject matter which the applicant regards as his invention. The test for definiteness asks whether one skilled in the art would understand the bounds of the claim when read in light of the specification... The level of skill assigned to a person of ordinary skill in the art... that is essential to administering the definiteness test... (is) a Bachelor's degree in a scientific or engineering field, such as physics, electrical engineering, or computer science, and at least two years of experience working in the field of computer telephony.. Claim definiteness, depends on the skill level of a person of ordinary skill in the art"*

"35 USC @112, para.1 *provides that the specification of a patent shall set forth the best mode contemplated by the inventor of carrying out his invention. This requirement ensures a patent applicant discloses the preferred embodiment of his invention. The purpose of the best mode requirement is to restrain inventors from applying for patents while at the same time concealing from the public preferred embodiments of the inventions they have in fact conceived... It is concealment of the best mode of practicing the* *claimed invention that is designed to prohibit... To apply the best mode standard, .. first determine whether, at the time the patent application was filed, the inventor had a best mode of practicing the claimed invention. This determination turns on the **inventor's own subjective beliefs**. The second part of the analysis* [asks] *... has the inventor 'concealed' his preferred mode from the 'public'?"*

(vii)  On October 27, 2009, Mr.Swift, Esq. and I met examiner Gilbert, and supervisor-Examiner Marmor; I presented that my method with 2-prongs, the *process* and the teaching, satisfies all the requirements of 35 USC @ 101 & 112, because-

**. the *process* part transforms brain-neurons into a different state for a specific purpose, and the teaching part enables one in the skill of the art understand the bounds of my claim.**

Then, Mr.Marmor/Gilbert gave me a copy of a memorandum dated August 24, 2009-

*'New Interim Patent Subject Matter Eligibility Examination Instructions'* (under 35 USC @101) *supersede previous guidance on the subject matter eligibility that conflicts with the instructions*, including MPEP 2106(IV), 2106.01 and 2106.02.

And, pointing to a sentence on page 5 (Exhibit 3.5)-

*"**Purely mental processes in which thoughts or human based actions are 'changed' are not considered an eligible transformation**"*, informed me of their inability to accept my method because of that *new* rule. They assured me <u>no</u> other examiner would be able to do any better either because Commissioner (Stoll) and others are aware of this *new* rule and my method...

(viii)  Therefore, on October 28-29, 2009 (Exhibit 3.6), I petitioned Commissioner Stoll seeking to 'invoke supervisory authority' in the matter [rule 181(3)]; and, spoke to Mr.Hejec (and Ms.Angela) in the Commissioner's office.

Mr.Hejec suggested I take an appeal before the Board upon receiving a final rejection from Mr.Gilbert; but, Commissioner Stoll did not respond to my petition.

(ix) Since 2006, USPTO's *in-house authority* discriminated me and my method in favor of pills or drugs abusing discretion; then, in August 2009 made effective a *new* rule keeping my patent application in a cold-storage (for nearly a year); and did not give me an opportunity to participate in this *new* rule making.

(x) USPTO's *in house authority* knowingly incorporated '*one-sentence substantive*' rule in the interim guidance to stop me from getting Patent, and give a free hand to the drug-makers. Thus, USPTO clearly violated my right to due process under 5 USCS §553(a)(2), (c) & (e) by refusing to consider my petition for amendment, or repeal of that '*one-sentence substantive*' rule.

**3.** *Undisputed* material-facts in *support* of my claim under APA@553 & 706.

(i)   On October 27, 2008, attorney Swift *re*-filed my Patent-application at No.12/259,285, a CiP2, consisting of a '*process with bands*'; because, on September 24, 2008, supervisor-Examiner Marmor rejected "*sleep study* (as) *likely not be useful*" and the "*pending method claims involve merely mental steps and are un-patentable and non-statutory*" (Exhibit 2.4).

(ii)  On September 26, 2009 (a year later…), examiner Gilbert's non-final rejection (Exhibit 3.4 on p.4-5) said-

Claim Rejections- 35 USC @ 101- "*Claims 1-20 are rejected under 35 USC 101 because the disclosed invention is inoperative and therefore lacks utility… In the instant case the process functions to change the processing of the brain. However it is examiner's position that changing the processing in the brain does not transform the brain… The activity caused by the method, 'cause the brain to produce melatonin' and 'helping the brain produce serotonin' are natural functions of the brain and therefore the brain has not been transformed only initiated to perform a function the brain normally performs. Therefore the claim is not directed to statutory subject matter*".

(iii) USPTO thru examiner Gilbert took that position '*in excess of statutory authority*' knowing 35 USC 101 (or Congress..) did <u>not</u> provide for '*at-will rejection* by *taking any position under the sun*', discarding-

(1) facts in my application that ".. *the split brain transforms brain-neurons into a different-physical state to flip off the light switch in the brain-stem. The brain having been repaired and transformed produces melatonin*", and

(2) the finding from a study at U. of Wisconsin "*meditation not only changes the working of the brain in the short term, but also quite possibly produces permanent changes...*"

(iv) Examiner Gilbert's rejection in 2009 is identical to that of a Jr.-Examiner's in 2007 (working for Pezzuto) who acted per the *dictates* of *in-house authority*. The only difference being the *dictates* in 2006-9 came in the absence of an 'Interim Guidance..', and by August 24, 2009, USPTO could create a change in policy to help justify the *old* and *new dictates* using or misusing <u>Bilski</u>...

(v) At the Interview on October 27, 2009, examiners gave me a copy of the document '*Interim Examination Instructions for Evaluating Subject Matter Eligibility under 35 USC 101*' (hereafter called 'Interim Guidance') which is made **effective on August 24, 2009**; and, pointed out to me (on p.5) that-

'*Purely mental processes in which thoughts or human based actions are "changed" are not considered an eligible transformation*'.

(vi) Examiner affirmed his rejection on the basis of this Interim Guidance, and expressed his inability to do any better on my application, or no other examiner can either. I thanked the examiners and left.

(vii)  On October 28, 2009, examiner Gilbert issued an Interview Summary (Exhibit 3.7), a copy of which Mr.Swift mailed to me on December 19, 2009; and it confirms the substance of examiner's rejection of my Patent-

*"The examiner took the position that the process is not statutory because '**Purely mental processes in which thoughts or human based actions are "changed" are not considered an eligible transformation**', page 5 of the 'Interim Examination Instructions for Evaluating Subject Matter Eligibility under 35 USC 101 '".*

(viii)  Until I received USPTO's motion to dismiss this action on or about March 31, 2010, I am not aware of the publication of a Notice under @ 553(c) on 'Interim Guidance'; and, no one informed me of that either at the Interview on October 27, 2009, or at any time before or after.

(ix)  On October 28-29, 2009 (Exhibit 3.6), I promptly submitted my comments, suggestions or objections based on the substance of examiner's rejection and USPTO's change in policy that it-

**"affirms prior-practice of discrimination against '*mental-process*', a judicially recognized exception, which is central to the purpose of the method I invented; and, the *mental process* in my method is limited to making *neurons* (specific to brain) attain a *different-state* or reduce to an active-state in producing melatonin-serotonin for the sleep-cycle** (*a particular practical application*). Sec 101"

I submitted my comments by facsimile to 571 273 0125 marked to the attention of the Commissioner on October 28-29, 2009, well before the deadline date of November 9, 2009.

(x)  Although the Notice advised that *"the USPTO will revise the* (Interim Guidance) *instructions as appropriate based on comments received"*, I did not receive any response to my comments from the Commissioner other than a suggestion (on phone from Mr.Hejec... as if the final-rejection is on the way) that I *take an appeal to the Board*.

(xi) USPTO did <u>not</u> notify me (or my Patent-attorney) on-

(1) its "*..consideration of the relevant matter presented*" by me or whether it "*incorporate*(d) *in the rule adopted* (which affected my rights) *a concise general statement of the basis and purpose*" under @553(c); and,

(2) whether its "*required publication or service of substantive rule is made not less than 30 days before effective date*" under @ 553(d); and,

(3) whether it "*..gave an interested person* (in this case…to me) *the right to petition for the issuance, amendment, or repeal of a rule*" as required under @ 553(e).

(xii) Thus, USPTO failed-

(1) to notify me of any amendment in policy or *repeal* of that '*one-sentence substantive*' rule'which affected my rights under @ 553, and

(2) to act on my Patent-application despite a timely response on December 23, 2009 (Exhibit 3.7.1) to examiner Gilbert's rejections.

USPTO's failure is arbitrary, capricious, and an abuse of discretion or otherwise not in accordance with law; or contrary to constitutional right, power, privilege, or immunity; or in excess of statutory jurisdiction, authority or limitations; and without observance of procedure required by law- under @ 706(2)(A), (B), (C), (D).

(xiii) Based on the facts known to me as of December 9, 2009, I originally commenced this action in USDC/DC at No.09-2417; on 12/21/09, judge of USDC/DC dismissed without prejudice my action as the "*venue in this case lies in the ED of Virginia and not with this court*".

(xiv) On December 24, 2009, I re-filed the same complaint with an application seeking leave to file.. in USDC/ED of Va. at No.09cv1412.

Thereafter, I contacted USPTO in an attempt to settle this matter amicably…promptly in the interest of the Public.

**4.** Issue(s) for *Review* by Fed.Cir.:

A. Judge Brinkema in her order of 30th April 2010 (DE 25) said-

*"For the reasons stated in open court, defendant's motion to dismiss is granted and plaintiff's motion to set aside USPTO's substantive rule… is denied, and, …ordered that this civil action …is dismissed with prejudice."*

And,

In the open court (per the court-transcript- DE 27) the judge stated-

*"As the government has correctly pointed out, you have not yet had a final agency action. ..by filing this lawsuit,.. you stopped that process, and… without a final action from the agency, you really have no basis to be in this court"* (p7, L18-24).

*"… under concepts of due process,.. there's absolutely nothing in your case to indicate.. anything amiss in how the matters have been handled. ..so under the Administrative Procedures Act, there really is nothing for this court to be looking at, and even if there were, the particular type of agency action about which you are ultimately complaining, …has to be addressed to one of two other courts"* (p.8, L18-25 & p.9 L1-3).

**Issue 1**:  Did the judge *abuse* power- to deny my request to set aside USPTO's "*substantive-rule*" under APA @553 & 706(2) and dismiss with "*prejudice*" my claim against USPTO- with a finding that the

*"Government has correctly pointed out I have not yet had a final agency action, and by filing the lawsuit (I) stopped that process, and without a final action (I) really have no basis to be in the court.. and there is absolutely nothing in (my) case to indicate anything amiss in how the matters have been handled (by USPTO) under the APA"*

**Answer-** Yes, the judge *abused* power due to her bias in favor of the government and prejudice against me (and 35% of the American People who suffer or face death with sleep-problems), and used or misused USPTO's *false*-arguments in its brief and at the hearing-

(i)  to <u>deny</u> a hearing on the *merits* or allow me present evidence on my claim under APA, and not allow discovery;

(ii)  to discard *undisputed* material facts in the record and *relevant*-law, and conclude that I "*stopped the process, and without a final action* (by USPTO on my patent) I *really have no basis to be in the court.. and there is absolutely nothing in* my *case to indicate anything amiss in how the matters have been handled* (by USPTO) *under the APA*"; and

(iii)  to "*grant*" government's motion to dismiss, and "*deny*" my motion to set aside USPTO's "*substantive*" rule and order that my action is "*dismissed with prejudice*", refusing to help *settle* the matter in the interest of 35% of the Public who suffer with sleep-problems…

B.  The judge in her order of May 18, 2010 (DE 33) said-

"*Mikkilineni has filed a motion for re-hearing on the merits… (and) has not pointed to any change in controlling law, new evidence not previously available, or any clear error of law… accordingly, plaintiff's motion to reconsider be and is denied*"

**Issue 2**:  Did the judge *err*- to deny my request for a re-*hearing* on the *merits* knowing she made APA @553 & 706(2) and the law of USSC & Fed.Cir. a "*dead letter*" ?

**Answer-** Yes, the judge *erred* in-

(iv)  discarding USSC & Fed.Cir. law to make APA @553 & 706(2) a "*dead letter*"…

**5.**  *Undisputed* material-facts and *relevant*-law in support of my **Answers**:

**_Issue_ 1**: Abuse of power

(i)  USPTO did <u>not</u> dispute any of the material-facts I stated or cited at **2** & **3**, above; but, it argued in its brief of April 21, 2010 (DE 21) that-

_"Plaintiff now asks this court to wade into the uncertain waters of substantive patent law_ (which are likely to change any day with the issuance of USSC's decision in <u>Bilski</u>), _and to do so within the context of his own specific patent application- which remains pending with USPTO at this time, and with respect to which plaintiff retains significant administrative and judicial review rights (p.3-4)… Congress has provided a comprehensive and mandatory scheme… that a patent applicant is required to await a final rejection of his application by an examiner, and appeal that decision to the Board, before seeking judicial review in an Article III court (p.9)… Congress, as a result of this exclusive scheme, has precluded a patent applicant from seeking generic judicial review of agency's patentability decisions under the APA outside of the scheme itself… (or) this court cannot exercise APA jurisdiction to review examiner's non-final rejection…(p.10)"_

_"Plaintiff attempts…to argue that a single sentence in USPTO's interim guidance serves as a substantive rule…because it substantively deprives his rights (p.5)… Perhaps more importantly, the interim guidance does not control the ultimate administrative or judicial decision concerning whether plaintiff's application is approved, and therefore cannot deprive plaintiff of any substantive rights under the Patent Act (p.7)… As such, even were USPTO examiners bound by the interim guidance, because the courts are not so bound, plaintiff's purported rights to patent his sleep method are not ultimately impacted by the interim guidance… if plaintiff's patent application is finally rejected by USPTO, he will…be entitled to present his views…to a specifically designated federal court without being hampered by the interim guidance (p.8)"_

Judge's bias in favor of the government and prejudice against me made her take sides with USPTO and use its _false_-arguments at a hearing on April 30, 2010, and not allow me *speak* or *respond* to any of the issues presented by USPTO; nor allowed me to *present* my motion to *set aside* the *substantive* rule- see transcript (DE 27). Judge did *not* even allow *discovery* or help settle the matter which I requested in the interest of nearly 35% of the American People who suffer with sleep-problems; and, judge denied a hearing on the *merits* or not allowed me present evidence on my claim under APA. Instead, the judge let USPTO place more *false*-arguments in the record on lack of *"final rejection"* of my patent and my *"ability to appeal"* to the Board and Fed.Cir. or USDC/DC (p.3, L24)- although the *final rejection* or my *ability to appeal* is not *relevant* to my pending claim under 5 USC @ 553 & 706(2).

(ii) Judge discarded *undisputed* material facts-

In May 2007, Mr.Swift and I met Mr.Pezzuto, supervisor-Examiner who informed that he is going to *"discuss with in-house authority"* as to the rejection under 35 USC @101 and, later he indicated likelihood of granting Patent- but, in October 2007, sent a **final** rejection per the *dictates* of *in-house authority*. In December 2007, I filed another application, CiP1. In June 2008, examiner Gilbert sent claim rejections (non-final) under 35 USC @101, *as non-statutory subject matter*; and under 35 USC @112 paras. 1-2, *as failing to comply with enablement requirement and as being indefinite claim…*, as before.

In August 2008, I met examiner Gilbert and explained how any one who is interested in the skill can be trained to use my method for beneficial use. Mr.Gilbert understood and his interview summary stated-

*"Mr.Mikkilineni explained that his method was not concentrating on a scene with two elements of an image at the same time, but, keep two separate elements as two separate thoughts,* (and) *bring them into the mind at the same time"*.

I also made it clear that a specification or a book can't teach some-one to ride a bike, or an MD-trainee do brain-Surgery on the first-day without proper training...; and if books can enable an ordinary skilled to do it, there is no need for teaching schools.

In September 2008, I had a telephone interview with supervisor-Examiner Marmor, and his summary says-

*"applicant explained... and suggested a sleep study be conducted to address the rejections... examiner explained that the sleep study would likely **not be useful**... that the pending method claims involve **merely mental steps** and are unpatentable and **nonstatutory**. A patent eligible process under 35 USC 101 must be tied to another statutory class, such as a particular apparatus, or **transform** underlying subject matter or material"*.

This is the same *dictates* the *in-house authority* kept giving to the examiners since 2006, knowing- my method administers electrical signals into a sick human brain, a physical object which contains neurons- physical substance, and help transform the neurons (that stopped working) into a different state to enable them work and produce melatonin and serotonin for a sleep cycle.

In October 2008, Mr.Swift, Esq., patent-attorney, filed a new application, CiP2; and, in September 2009, I discovered an article published in Washington Post titled '*Meditation Gives Brain a Charge*...'- a study conducted at U. of Wisconsin with the help of **Dalai Lama** (the study-results were published in American National Academy of Science Journal);  I forwarded that to examiner Gilbert.

After seeing that evidence, on October 01, 2009, examiner Gilbert sent a non-final *rejection* under 35 USC @101, as *inoperative and lacks utility*; and under 35 USC @112 paras. 1-2, as failing to comply with *enablement requirement* and as being *indefinite* claim etc.., as before.  As stated above, in September 2008, the *in-house authority* stopped me from undertaking a '*sleep study*' to show the method works for a useful result; and in October 2009 rejects the method as '*inoperative and lacks utility*', asserting its right to take any position under the sun- "*it is examiner's position that.. the processing in the brain does not transform the brain*"

I did not make the claim that my *process* "*transforms the brain*"- I claimed my *process transforms the neurons into a different state to enable them produce melatonin and serotonin*... So, clearly, the *in house authority* is either incompetent or arrogant with power over the People to think it can take any position under the sun... as no one is checking on them- see <u>Bilski</u> at 2006 WL 5738364 (on p.4), where the Board said-

*"Only a very small fraction of the cases examined by the Examining Corps are ever appealed to the Board, and only a very small fraction of the rejections affirmed by the Board will ever be appealed to the Fed.Cir...".*

Examiner Gilbert's rejection in 2009 is identical to that of a Jr.-Examiner's in 2007 (working for Pezzuto) per the *dictates* of *in-house authority*. The only difference being the *dictates* in 2006-9 came in the absence of an 'Interim Guidance..', and by August 24, 2009, USPTO could create a *substantive* rule or change in policy to help justify the *old* and *new dictates* using or misusing <u>Bilski</u>...

At the Interview on October 27, 2009, examiners gave me a copy of the document '*Interim Examination Instructions for Evaluating Subject Matter Eligibility under 35 USC 101*' (hereafter called 'Interim Guidance') which is made **effective on August 24, 2009**; and, pointed out to me (on p.5) that-

'*Purely mental processes in which thoughts or human based actions are "changed" are not considered an eligible transformation*'.

Examiners agreed the rejection is based on this Interim Guidance, and expressed inability to do any better on my application, or no other examiner can either. Therefore, on October 28-29, 2009, I promptly submitted my comments, suggestions or objections based on the substance of examiner's rejection and USPTO's change in policy-

**"affirms prior-practice of discrimination against '*mental-process*', a judicially recognized exception, which is central to the purpose of the method I invented; and, the *mental process* in my method is**

**limited to making *neurons* (specific to brain) attain a *different-state* or reduce to an active-state in producing melatonin-serotonin for the sleep-cycle** (*a particular practical application*). Sec 101"

Later, examiner Gilbert issued an Interview Summary (Exhibit 3.7), a copy of which Mr.Swift mailed to me on December 19, 2009, which confirms the substance of examiner's rejection of my Patent-

*"The examiner took the position that the process is not statutory because '**Purely mental processes in which thoughts or human based actions are "changed" are not considered an eligible transformation**', page 5 of the 'Interim Examination Instructions for Evaluating Subject Matter Eligibility under 35 USC 101 '".*

Until I received USPTO's motion to dismiss this action on or about March 31, 2010, I am not aware of the publication of a Notice on 'Interim Guidance' under @553(c); and, <u>no one</u> informed me of that either at the Interview on October 27, 2009, or at any time before or after. However, by chance, my comments to the Commissioner by facsimile (at 571 273 0125) on October 28-29, 2009, are sent before the deadline date of November 9, 2009.

Although the Notice advised that *"the USPTO will revise the* (Interim Guidance) *instructions as appropriate based on comments received"*, I did <u>not</u> receive any response to my comments from the Commissioner other than a suggestion (on phone from Mr.Hejec… as if the final-rejection is on the way) that I *take an appeal to the Board.*

USPTO did <u>not</u> notify me (or my Patent-attorney) on-

. its *"..consideration of the relevant matter presented"* by me or whether it *"incorporate*(d) *in the rule adopted* (which affected my rights) *a concise general statement of the basis and purpose"* as required under @ 553(c); and,

. whether its *"required publication or service of substantive rule is made not less than 30 days before effective date"* under @ 553(d); and,

. whether it "*..gave an interested person* (in this case…to me) *the right to petition for the issuance, amendment, or repeal of a rule*" as required under @ 553(e).

Thus, USPTO failed-

to notify me of amendment to policy or *repeal* of that '*one-sentence substantive*' rule which affected my rights under @ 553, and

. to act on my Patent-application despite a timely response on December 23, 2009 (Exhibit 3.7.1) to examiner Gilbert's rejections.

For that reason, USPTO's failure is arbitrary, capricious, and an abuse of discretion or otherwise not in accordance with law; or contrary to constitutional right, power, privilege, or immunity; or in excess of statutory jurisdiction, authority or limitations; and without observance of procedure required by law- under @ 706(2)(A), (B), (C), (D).

Judge discarded *relevant*-law of USSC & Fed.Cir. and made APA a '*dead letter*'(see DE 15-16 & 23)-

In this process of choosing sides, the judge did not bother even to look into the key-issue I raised- because USPTO did not want her to address it:

Whether USPTO '*failed to take a discrete action*', it is required to take upon receiving my timely comments and repeal the '*substantive*' rule made effective on August 24, 2009, before notice and public comment-

The policy USPTO used against me for nearly 4-years, *first* through the '*in-house authority*' in the absence of a formal change in the rule, and *now* with an official-change in the policy, which made my compliance essentially impossible and substantively deprived my rights under APA- 5 USC @ 553(c), (d) & (e), and 706(2).

See Norton, 542 US 55, USSC said:

*"The Administrative Procedure Act (APA) authorizes suit by a person suffering legal wrong because of agency action, or adversely affected or aggrieved by agency action within the meaning of a relevant statute. 5 USC 702. Where no other statute provides a private right of action, the agency action complained of must be final agency action. 5 USC 704. Agency action is defined in 5 USC 551(13) to include **the whole or a part of an agency rule**, order **or the equivalent or denial thereof, or failure to act**.*

*The final term in the definition set forth in 5 USC 551(13), "**failure to act**," is properly understood **as a failure to take an agency action**; that is, a failure to take one of the agency actions (including their equivalents) earlier defined in 551(13). For purposes of 5 USC 551(a), a failure to act is not the same thing as a denial. The latter is the agency's act of saying no to a request; the former is **simply the omission of an action without formally rejecting a request**, for example, the failure to promulgate a rule or take some decision by a statutory deadline. The important point is that a "failure to act" is properly understood to be limited, as are the other items in 551(13), to a **discrete action**. The only agency action that can be compelled under the Administrative Procedure Act is action legally required...A claim under 5 USC 706(1) can proceed only where a plaintiff **asserts that an agency failed to take a discrete agency action that it is required to take... Unless and until the (agency act) is amended, such actions can be set aside as contrary to law pursuant to 5 USC 706(2)".***

See Cooper, 536 F.3d 1330 (2008), Fed Cir. said-

*"We have also previously held that 35 USC @ 2(b)(2) does not authorize the Patent Office to issue "substantive" rules. See Merck, 80 F.3d 1543. "A rule is 'substantive' when it 'effects a change in existing law or policy' which 'affect[s] individual rights and obligations." Animal, 932 F.2d at 927. "In contrast, a rule which merely clarifies or explains existing law or regulations is 'interpretative."*

And, in <u>Tafas</u>, 559 F.3d 1345 (2009), Fed. Cir. (*en banc*) analyzed the distinction between '*substantive*' and procedural (or *interpretive*) rule-making by USPTO, and said-

"*While the text of the rules sets forth a facially reasonable procedural requirement, we are mindful of the possibility that the USPTO may in some cases attempt to apply the rules in a way that makes compliance essentially impossible and substantively deprives applicants of their rights. In such cases, judicial review will be available under* <u>5 USC @ 706</u>". In <u>Animal</u>, 932 F.2d 920 "*To establish standing to sue, a party must, at an irreducible minimum, show* (1) *that he personally has suffered some actual or threatened injury as a result of the putatively illegal conduct* (personal injury), (2) *that the injury fairly can be traced to the challenged action* (causation), *and* (3) *that the injury is likely to be redressed by a favorable decision* (effective relief). *In addition to these requirements, standing is further limited to those parties within the "zone of interests" a particular statute addresses*" (35 USC @ 101...)

That's precisely what USPTO did here using the exception under @ 553(b)(A) made effective on **August 24, 2009** an Interim Guidance…that contained at least *one-substantive* rule to apply in a way that makes my compliance essentially impossible and substantively deprives my right. So, in this case *judicial review* is *available under* <u>5 USC @ 706</u>, because under the guise of an '*interpretive*' rulemaking USPTO effectively put out an Interim Guidance that included a '*substantive*' rule-

**"*Purely mental processes in which thoughts or human based actions are 'changed' are not considered an eligible transformation*"**.

<u>No</u> court in the land has <u>ever</u> said "*mental processes in which thoughts or human based action*-changes.. *are not considered an eligible transformation*"; USPTO's *in-house authority* simply made this up…as if they can take '*any position under the sun…*' This is a change in the existing law or policy as it impermissibly substantive, inconsistent with law, arbitrary and capricious, incomprehensibly vague, impermissibly retroactive, and procedurally defective, and affects my individual rights

and obligations under Bilski. In Bilski, 545 F.3d 943 (2008), Fed Cir. (*en banc*) analyzed whether a claim reciting *mental process* is drawn to patent-eligible subject matter under 35 USC @ 101, an issue of law, and said (in judges' own words)-

*"..we address a possible misunderstanding of our decision in Comiskey. Some may suggest that Comiskey implicitly applied a new @ 101 test that bars any claim reciting a mental process that lacks significant "physical steps." We did not so hold, nor did we announce any new test at all in Comiskey. Rather, we simply recognized that the Supreme Court has held that mental processes, like fundamental principles, are excluded by @ 101 because "'[p]henomena of nature, though just discovered, mental processes, and abstract intellectual concepts . . . are the basic tools of scientific and technological work.'" Comiskey, 499 US at 1377… Because those claims failed the machine-or-transformation test, we held that they were drawn solely to a fundamental principle, the mental process of arbitrating a dispute, and were thus not patent-eligible under @ 101.*

*… when the claim at issue recites fundamental principles other than mathematical algorithms… the proper inquiry under @ 101 is not whether the process claim recites sufficient "physical steps," but rather whether the claim meets the machine-or-transformation test. As a result, even a claim that recites "physical steps" but neither recites a particular machine or apparatus, nor transforms any article into a different state or thing, is not drawn to patent-eligible subject matter. Conversely, a claim that purportedly lacks any "physical steps" but is still tied to a machine or achieves an eligible transformation passes muster under @ 101".*

Fed Cir. in conclusion, also said- *"Of course, a claimed process wherein all of the process steps may be performed entirely in the human mind is obviously not tied to any machine and **does not transform any article into a different state or thing**. As a result, it would not be patent-eligible under @ 101".*

By that Fed. Cir. can only mean **if** *"…process steps performed entirely in the human mind **does not transform** any article* or substance out-side of "brain" *into a different state*" **it would not be patent-eligible** under @ 101; but, per USPTO **if** "**mental processes in which thoughts or human based actions** (cause) **changes** in the "brain-neurons", (such changes) **are not considered an eligible transformation".** Clearly, this is a new *substantive* rule or change in the policy, a *substantive* change; and <u>Bilski</u> or the Congress did not give that power to USPTO. It simply assumed that power to create the law on its own using or misusing <u>Bilski</u> and discriminated my method which is based on '*mental process*'. After losing 4- years in trying to persuade USPTO to issue Patent, now, it appears I have to spend several years more in appeals, if I can at 71, and being a recovered *leukemia* patient…

(iii)  Contrary to the *undisputed* material facts and *relevant* law cited, the judge concludes that-

I "*stopped the process, and without a final action* (by USPTO on my patent) I *really have no basis to be in the court… and there is absolutely nothing in* my *case to indicate anything amiss in how the matters have been handled* (by USPTO) *under the APA*"

And, "*granted*" government's motion to dismiss my claim under APA, and "*denied*" my motion to set aside USPTO's "*substantive*" rule, and on her own motion ordered that my action is "*dismissed with prejudice*" refusing to help *settle* the matter in the interest of nearly 35% of the American People who suffer with sleep-problems or the drugs.. (including facing death like Michael Jackson).

*Issue* 2:  Judge *erred* in-

(iv)  discarding USSC & Fed.Cir. law to make APA @553 & 706(2) a "*dead letter*"

At the hearing on April 30, 2010 (see transcript DE 27), judge's line of inquiry is clearly intended to make APA a '*dead letter*' and thrash USSC & Fed.Cir. law and a recent ruling in <u>Commonwealth</u> v. US, 2009 US Dist. LEXIS 110293 (2009) where judge Friedman of USDC/DC said-

*"A party experiences actionable harm when "depriv[ed] of a procedural protection to which he is entitled" under the APA.* <u>Sugar Cane Growers</u>, 289 F.3d 89. *If such were not the case, "*<u>sec. 553</u> *would be a dead letter." If defendants have in fact violated the APA's notice-and-comment provisions, then, there is no question that the (plaintiff) will be injured by the implementation of the Interim... Rule.*

Judge says *"by filing this complaint, under the Patent Office's practice, stopped.. evaluation..."*; and USPTO responds- *"when an Article III case is filed regarding a particular patent application,... they will stop prosecution ...That is not a hard-and-fast rule...they have applied that rule in this context"* (p.4, L1-12).

<u>Response</u>: Whether or not my claim under APA is an Article III case, USPTO has absolutely *no*-authority under the statute to make-up a *"rule"* to stop evaluation of my pending patent-application since December 2009 [see at **3**(xii)(2)].

Judge says *".. the interpretive guidance* (USPTO) *issued while they await the Supreme Court to resolve or... address Fed. Cir.'s latest ruling on method..(in Bilski)"*; and USPTO responds- USPTO *"made very clear that because it is an interpretive rule, it's not substantive rule making..."* (p.4, L15-24).

<u>Response</u>: The *undisputed* material facts I stated [see at **3**(i)-(xii)] makes absolutely clear that under the guise of interpretive rules USPTO included at least *'one substantive-rule'* and deprived my rights...

Judge concludes *"the way law is set up, this court and no Article III court has the ability to rewrite the interpretive rules"* of USPTO; and USPTO responds- *"That's correct"* (p.5, L7-10).

<u>Response</u>: My pending-claim in this action under 5 USC @706(2) is not *"to rewrite the interpretive rules"*, but *"to set aside that one sentence substantive rule"*, that USPTO has used or misused against me during the past 4-years depriving me of my rights, and thus negligently caused injury to about 35% of the Americans who are

suffering with insomnia or the drugs (or even face-*death* like Michael Jackson).

Judge raises the issue of *"proper procedure… due process issue… failure to provide notice…"*; and USPTO agrees *"the Fed. Cir… has the authority to tell USPTO that its interpretive guidance is wrong"* (p.5, L12-3 & L19-21).

Judge says *"On the merits"*; and USPTO agrees *"correct"* (p.5, L22-3).

<u>Response</u>: Although the court has the ability under 5 USC @706(2) *to set aside a substantive rule…*, the judge did *not* go into the *merits* knowing it is her *duty* to get to the '*merits*' in this case before making conclusions…..

Judge concludes *"It's not an abstract process where there's been no final rejection…"* (p.6, L22-3); and USPTO says- *"there would be no standing for an individual…unless there was some reasonable expectation that it would be applied against them in a detrimental way…"* (p.7, L1-3).

<u>Response</u>: I made that absolutely clear in the facts and in my briefs that the issue of '*final rejection*' is a *non-issue* under 5 USC @553 & 706(2), because my claim is based on USPTO's *use or misuse of a new substantive rule against me in a detrimental way…*

Then, the judge tells me-

*"the reality of it is that the lawsuit that you have filed in this court and the motion…, have no legal foundation. As the government has correctly pointed out, you have not yet had a final agency action… patent has not finally been rejected… by filing this lawsuit, basically you stopped that process… without a final action from the agency, you really have no basis to be in this court (p.7, L12-24)… All we would be concerned… is whether the process was appropriate… under concepts of due process,…, there's absolutely nothing in your case to indicate that there's been anything amiss in how the matters have been handled (p.8, L16-21)…. For these reasons defendant's motion*

*to dismiss is granted. This case is dismissed. Your motion to set aside the substantive rule is denied* (p.9, L6-8)."

*Response*: But, the order of 30th April 2010, says- "*defendant's motion to dismiss is granted and plaintiff's motion to set aside PTO's substantive rule & declaratory order is denied... this civil action is dismissed with **prejudice**...*" USPTO did *not* ask my case be "*dismissed with prejudice*", the judge did so on her own motion contrary to her own proclamation in the open court- "*this case is dismissed*" (p.9, L7). In doing so, the judge did <u>not</u> even consider to help <u>settle</u> the issue amicably despite my request... And, the order is made with '*bias and prejudice*', against me and other 35% of Americans with an out-right *denial* of a hearing on the *merits*. Thus, not *only* USPTO denied due process, but the judge too *did* the same by accepting USPTO's *false*-arguments....and in the process bypassed the key-issue needed to be decided-

"Whether USPTO has '*failed to take a discrete action*', which is required to take upon receiving my timely comments, and repeal the '*substantive*' rule or change in policy made effective on August 24, 2009, before notice and public comment under APA @ 553(c), (d) & (e), and 706(2)". <u>Norton</u>, 542 US 55; <u>Tafas</u>, 559 F.3d 1345.

On May 18, 2010 (DE 33), the judge <u>denied</u> my motion for a *re-*hearing on the merits (May 17, 2010: DE 20-30) by misusing 4th Cir. law. See <u>Ingle</u>, 439 F.3d 191 ("*motion will be granted in three circumstances: (1) to accommodate an intervening change in controlling law; (2) to account for new evidence not available at trial; or (3) to correct a clear error of law or prevent manifest injustice*"). The judge knew she (1) '*discarded*' the controlling law of USSC & Fed.Cir. to thrash APA @553 & 706 as a "*dead letter*"; (2) '*discarded*' the *undisputed* material facts and refused to allow discovery; or (3) made a clear *error* of law (abusing discretion) and caused manifest injustice to nearly 35% of the American People by taking sides with USPTO...

**6.** *Action* Fed.Cir. *can Take*:

I request the Honorable judges to help settle *amicably* on the issue of *'substantive'* rule which USPTO has used or misused against me and my method *in a detrimental way*; or set aside the *'one-sentence substantive'* rule; or remand the case to the judge with instructions to set aside that *new*-rule under @706(2) and enter a declaratory order (per my motion DE 15).

Respectfully,
M.R.Mikkilineni
PO Box 32110
Washington, DC 20007

I certify that I hand delivered a copy of this pleading on June 15, 2010 to the office of US attorney ED of Va. at- US attorney, 2100 Jamieson Ave., Alexandria, Va. 22314

**UNITED STATES COURT OF APPEALS for the** Federal Cir.

No. 2010-1362

M.R.Mikkilineni
                Plaintiff-Appellant,
v.

Robert STOLL, Commissioner for Patents,
                Defendant-Appellee.

Appeal from the United States District Court for the Eastern District of Virginia, Case No. 09-cv-1412, Judge Leonie M. Brinkema.


*Informal* **Reply Brief to Appellee's** out of time *Brief*

Facts *relevant* to Appellee's *Brief*:

1. Clerk of this court docketed my appeal on 05/25/2010 with a critical date set for entry of appearance to be within 14 days from 05/25/2010 (or by 06/08/2010).

(i) Clerk rejected Appellee's entry of appearance dated 06/10/2010, and on 06/17/2010 Appellee amended entry without a motion to do so.

2. The critical date set under this Court's rule for filing my brief (informal) is within 21 days from 05/25/2010 (or by 06/15/2010).

(i) I filed my brief timely and on 06/15/2010, personally served a copy upon Dennis Barghaan (attorney of record for the Commissioner); and my certificate of service confirms that.

3. The critical date set under this Court's rule for filing Appellee's brief (formal) is within 40 days from 06/15/2010 (or by 07/26/2010). See Exb. 4.

(i) Appellee submitted its brief on 07/28/2010 (2-days too late), without a motion for 'leave of court' required under the rule for filing out of time; then, on 07/29/2010, clerk rejected that brief wanting a 'table of content' and ordered Appellee to file a 'corrected version' within 14 days...

4. In the Brief for Appellee (p.19- foot note) said-

*"On July 27, 2010, the USPTO issued further guidance to supplement the Interim guidelines, in response to the Supreme Court's decision in Bilski...The Interim Bilski guidance noted that the USPTO* **'has received and considered the comments** *regarding the (Interim guidelines)* **submitted in response to'** *the request for comments..."*

(i) That shows Appellee for its own convenience disregarded the rules of this Court and waited until after July 27, 2010 to submit its brief out of time and without a motion for 'leave of court'.

(ii) In this *"Interim Bilski guidance"* (Exhibit 4.1), USPTO claims:

. *"This guidance supersedes previous guidance on subject matter eligibility that conflicts with the Interim Bilski guidance"* (on 43922);

. *"It is intended to be used by office personnel as a supplement to the previously issued Interim Examination Instructions for Evaluating Subject Matter Eligibility...@101 dated August 24, 2009"* (on 43923);

. *"This additional guidance, which builds upon the 2009 Interim Instructions, is a factor-based inquiry....Examiners will recognize that the machine-or-transformation test set forth in Sec. II(B) of the 2009 Interim Instructions, although not the sole test for evaluating the subject matter eligibility of a method claim, is still pertinent in making determinations pursuant to the factors...."* (on 43925).

(iii) A first look at (USPTO's) the wording that the Interim *Bilski* guidance *"supersedes previous guidance...."* appears as if the 'discriminatory-rule' (*Purely mental processes in which thoughts or human based actions changed are not considered an eligible transformation*) is abandoned (see my Brief Exhibit 3.5 or Appendix for Appellee A21).

(iv) A closer look at (USPTO's) other wording that it is a *"supplement to the previously issued...,* (or) *additional guidance which builds upon the 2009 Interim Instruction...,* (and) *test set forth in Sec. II(B)...is still pertinent in making determinations..."* makes it clear that the 'discriminatory-rule' against my method is still alive and active…

5. Also, USPTO claims that-

. it *"has received and considered the comments regarding the* (Interim guidelines of 2009) *submitted in response to the request for comments..."* (see at 4, above); and,

. *"the fact that Mikkilineni had an opportunity to comment on the Interim guidelines- both before and after the examiner issued an initial rejection of Mikkilineni's claims on October 27, 2009- but failed to do so undermines his current claim that the USPTO deprived him of any rights under the APA"* (Brief for Appellee p.13-4).

(i) In fact, USPTO did <u>not</u> consider my comments of October 29, 2009 (see Exhibit 3.6 attached to my Brief) which I submitted by fax within the deadline set for November 9, 2009 (A48).

6. On 08/02/2010, I renewed my efforts to see if this can be settled amicably; but, no progress is made (Exhibit 4.2).

(i) On 08/05/2010, I submitted comments to USPTO in response to its notice on Interim *Bilski* guidance of July 27, 2010; and, again, I asked USPTO to repeal that substantive and discriminatory rule in the Interim Instructions of 2009 (Exhibit 4.3).

<u>*Response* to Appellee's *Brief*</u>:

I. *Statement of the issue*: I had no choice, but, to file this suit under APA because of USPTO's failure to amend or repeal

that one-sentence substantive rule it included in the Interim Instructions of 2009 that- *"Purely mental processes in which thoughts or human based actions are changed are not considered an eligible transformation"*- and, its use or misuse against my method for 4 years: first through its in-house authority in the absence of a formal change in the rule, and then with an official change in the policy- making my compliance essentially impossible and substantively deprived my rights under APA @553 (c), (d) & (e) and @706(2). USPTO failed to take a discrete action which it is required to take upon receiving my timely comments; and, it refused to repeal the substantive rule which is made effective on August 24, 2009, before notice and public comment.

USDC/ED of Va. dismissed my suit claiming 'lack of jurisdiction' after refusing to consider merits of my claim under APA. The judge disregarded evidence in the record and refused to allow discovery. The judge did not decide whether or not the discriminatory rule is substantive; but, simply dismissed my claims under APA because

there is no final-rejection on my patent. As a matter of law whether or not there is a final-rejection on my patent by USPTO is not relevant to my claims or the jurisdiction of the court under APA. For that reason the judge's dismissal of my claims under APA is clearly an abuse of power, which this Court can set aside and remand the case with instructions for further proceedings....

II. *Statement of the case*: I originally filed this case on December 9, 2009 in USDC/DC; because of venue question, I had to re-file it on December 24, 2009 in USDC/ED of Va. My Complaint (A115-6 at 11) states-

*"Thus, USPTO clearly violated my right to due process under 5 USC @553(a)(2), (c) & (e) by refusing to consider my petition for amendment or repeal of that one-sentence in the new-rule"*.

USDC/ED of Va. disregarded my claim under APA because of my *pro se* status and considered APA as a *dead*-letter with respect to my

rights (and the rights of 35% of the other Americans…who need a 'sleep method', not drugs).

III. *Statement of the facts*: On September 26, 2009 (A77) USPTO rejected my method twisting evidence and said (A81)-

*"In the instant case the process functions to change the processing of the brain. However it is the examiner's position that changing the processing in the brain does not transform the brain…The activity caused by the method, cause the brain to produce melatonin and helping the brain produce serotonin are natural functions of the brain and therefore the brain has not been transformed only initiated to perform a function the brain normally performs. Therefore the claim is not directed to statutory subject matter."*

On October 27, 2009, at a meeting, the examiner gave me a copy of USPTO's Interim Instructions, which were made effective on August 24, 2009 (A16-26), and pointing to *"Purely mental processes in which thoughts or human based actions are changed are not considered an eligible transformation"* (A21) declined to re-consider his rejection of my method claims; no one has ever gave me the pages that appear in the Appendix for Appellee (A27-49).

Subsequently, the examiner issued a an Interview Summary (A92 or Exhibit 3.7) and said-

"The examiner took the position that the process is not statutory because *Purely mental processes in which thoughts or human based actions are changed are not considered an eligible transformation*"

Thus, the examiner simply closed the book on me by using or misusing that new-rule in the Interim Instructions of 2009, which USPTO set solely for the purpose of discriminating my method. Thereafter, USPTO failed to amend or repeal that discriminatory-rule despite my timely comments or objections of October 29, 2009 (Exhibit 3.6). Therefore, I had no choice, but to commence an action under APA on December 9, 2009 in USDC/DC or re-file it on December 24, 2009 in USDC/ED of Va.

Although on December 23, 2009, I filed a response to examiner's rejection with an evidentiary Affidavit (Exhibit 3.7.1), USPTO, on its own, chose not to act on my patent-application for nearly 8-months, like what it did before several years…

B. *USPTO's Interim Instructions*: Even if most of the other Interim Instructions of 2009 are not substantive, one new-rule that "*Purely mental processes in which thoughts or human based actions are changed are not considered an eligible transformation*" is substantive; because, no other court in the land has ever put such a limitation on patentability under @ 101, and in June 2010 the USSC clearly rejected the notion of such limitations in *Bilski* (see Exhibit 4.3). In fact, in my case, USPTO used or misused that substantive rule and made my compliance essentially impossible and substantively deprived my rights under APA @553 (c), (d) & (e) and @706(2). USPTO simply disregarded my timely comments or objections on this substantive rule and refused to amend or repeal it.

IV. *Summary of the argument*: USDC/ED of Va. did not rule whether "*Purely mental processes in which thoughts or human based actions are changed are not considered an eligible transformation*" is an interpretive or substantive rulemaking; it simply ducked the issue by going in the wrong-way taking US attorney's guidance, and dismissed my claims under APA for lack of jurisdiction using a pretext that USPTO has not made a final-rejection on my request for patent. See court transcript, DE27 on p.5, L22 & p.7, L18-24.

As stated, I did timely submit my comments or objections to the new substantive rule, but, USPTO failed to amend or repeal the new rule. Therefore, USDC/ED of Va. has jurisdiction to hear my claims under APA despite lack of final rejection of patent by USPTO; and final rejection of patent is not relevant for jurisdiction of the court under APA.

V. *Argument*: Although my complaint and pleadings alleged sufficient relevant facts with undisputed material evidence, and made arguments citing relevant law under APA, the judge decided to take the side of government using US attorney's false-arguments, and nothing-else mattered... to declare that USDC/ED of Va. lacked jurisdiction because USPTO has not made a final-rejection of my request for patent...

B. ...*Properly dismissed*...: As I stated above, the issue is not the notice or the opportunity to comment on USPTO's Interim Instructions of 2009; the issue is whether or not that one-sentence new-rule is substantive and whether or not USPTO failed to amend or repeal that new-rule despite my timely comments and misused that rule to deprive my rights under APA. The judge did not rule on this key issue.

Therefore, Appellee's argument on a *non*-issue that the one-sentence new-rule is interpretive is not relevant at this time. The only question this Court should resolve at this stage is- whether USDC/ED of Va. has jurisdiction in the matter under APA. If the answer is yes- this Court should vacate district court orders and remand the case with instructions for further proceedings...

For that reason, I need not respond to Appellee's other arguments at C.

Respectfully,

M.R.Mikkilineni
PO Box 32110
Washington, DC 20007

Certificate of Service

I certify that I served a copy of this pleading on August 6, 2010 by US mail to-

Mary Kelly, Esq
Office of the Solicitor, USPTO
PO Box 15667
Arlington, Va. 22215

**UNITED STATES COURT OF APPEALS** FOR THE FEDERAL Cir. No. 2010-1362

M.R.Mikkilineni
        Plaintiff-Appellant,
v.

Robert STOLL, Commissioner of Patents,
        Defendant-Appellee.

Appeal from the United States District Court for the Eastern District of Virginia, Case No. 09-cv-1412, Judge Leonie M. Brinkema.

***Informal*** Petition ***of Appellant*** for rehearing and rehearing ***en banc***

This court's notice of September 21, 2010 advised "*a review of this case indicates that oral argument is not required and that the appeal may be decided on the briefs without prejudice...*"

On November 9, 2010, a panel of this court chose two *non*-issues, neglecting the issues I raised, to decide in favor of USPTO. It is obvious, the way panel did, it has no interest in justice or unable to be "*fair*"- because, it is a *pro se* appeal- who cares. So, the panel decided to shield the US agents- knowing of their continued wrongful-acts for nearly 4½ years- by entering a "*nonprecedential*" opinion, only applicable to this *pro se*, and no one-else...(copy of opinion attached). Therefore, I ask for a "*fair*" rehearing before the panel and/or the *en banc* court for the reason given below:

*First*, the two *non*-issues panel picked are (1) whether the Interim Guidelines are substantive rules improperly promulgated without *notice and comment rulemaking*, and (2) whether USPTO examiner improperly rejected (the) application (for patent)-

The issues I raised in my appeal are (1) did the judge abuse power to deny my request to set aside USPTO's "*substantive rule*" under APA

@553 & 706(2)..., and (2) did the judge err to deny my request for a re-hearing on the merits knowing she made APA @553 & 706(2) and the law of USSC...a "*dead letter*"

I did not ask the panel to review the two *non*-issues it chose to decide in favor of USPTO. Those *non*-issues are the ones USPTO has used to divert the attention of both the judge and the panel away from its wrongful acts under APA. In fact, I have not claimed that all Guidelines are substantive and needed '*notice and comment rulemaking*'. I claimed that only one substantive *new*-rule is included in the guidelines, solely to discriminate my method. The judge did not decide whether that one *new*-rule, I complained about, is 'substantive' or 'interpretive'; therefore, panel has no jurisdiction to decide on issue (1) when the trial judge failed to make the finding or decide.

My complaint (see under jurisdiction) asserted a claim that USPTO violated 5 USC @553(e)- "*Agency shall give an interested person the right to petition for the issuance , amendment, or repeal of a rule*". That is the only issue under APA the trial-judge had jurisdiction to decide after finding of the facts. The judge did not claiming lack of jurisdiction without a final-rejection of patent in my case. The court record shows I timely submitted comments, not once, but more than twice, to USPTO on this one *new*-rule in its Guidelines- but USPTO failed to repeal that discriminatory substantive *new* rule which it included in the Guidelines under the guise of 'interpretive' guidance. See USPTO's deceitful notice that panel cites on p.3: "*examination instructions do not constitute substantive rule making and hence do not have the force and effect of law*". It is deceitful, because the judge and the panel knew (see court record) the examiner and USPTO has been using that discriminatory *new*-rule in my case, selectively, for years... and claims it "*do not have the force and effect of law*".

I have not, yet, asked the judge or the panel to review USPTO's '*improper*' rejection of my application for patent. I only asked the court to find if USPTO's that one *new*-rule or policy that "*purely mental processes in which thoughts or human based actions are 'changed' are not considered an eligible transformation*" made part of the interim Guidelines is substantive, and discriminated my method affecting my rights. The judge refused to make a finding on that and declared that the trial-court has no jurisdiction to hear the case under APA 'without a final-rejection of patent'.

*Second*, with the above relevant facts in hand let us look into panel's discussion:

The panel correctly stated the law (p.4) *"A rule is substantive where it causes a change in existing law or policy that affects individual rights and obligations and interpretive where it merely clarifies or explains existing law or regulation"*. But, it concluded on its own, in the absence of judge's finding- my showing that 'one *new*-rule in the Guidelines is substantive within the meaning of APA as it substantively deprived my rights', is *"without merit"*- because USPTO's guidelines are (1) *"based on the.. current understanding of the law"* and (2) *"do not have the force and effect of law"*.

The panel is incorrect on both fronts- because (1) no court in the land has ever made a law to enable USPTO come up with a *new*-rule and discriminate my method under the pretext *"current understanding of the law"*, and (2) alleged facts in my complaint and the court-record show USPTO used that *new*-rule against my method for 4½ years. It used that *new*-rule (thru examiners several times) and once even entered a *final*-rejection of patent; and, it is a repetition of the same act. So, USPTO's assertion that the *new*-rule has *"no force and effect of law"* is a deceit and fraud…., and Panel's theory (p.6) that *"Mikkilineni could still overcome the non-final rejection and receive a patent"* has no basis.

Then, panel says (p.4-5) *"our decision in* Animal… *is almost directly on point"*, because PTO's notice in Animal… *"mirrored the Supreme Court's holding in* Diamond…*"* So, *"this court rejected th*(at) *plaintiff's argument, finding that the USPTO notice was interpretive rather than substantive"*. Yes, makes sense in that case because USPTO's notice simply *"mirrored"* the law of the highest court in the land. In my case, there is no such law to mirror or enable USPTO discriminate at will. It simply made this *new*-rule to justify its wrongful-acts in my case since 2006, and stop me from obtaining a patent... It is that simple, and not hard to see the difference between that case in Animal... and the present case.

Finally, the panel says (p.5) *"we conclude that the Interim Guidelines are interpretive, rather than substantive, and are thus exempt from notice and comment..."* First, this case is not about all *"Guidelines"*, it is about one substantive *new*-rule USPTO included in the Guidelines to stop me from getting patent. Second, the panel has no jurisdiction to decide on an issue- whether or not that one *new*-rule is substantive- when the trial-judge did not rule on it.

Conclusion

For the reasons stated above, I request the *en banc* court to remand the case back to the trial-judge for a finding of the facts after allowing proper discovery.

Respectfully,

M.R.Mikkilineni
PO Box 32110
Washington, DC 20007

Certificate of Service

I certify that I served a copy of this pleading on November 17, 2010 by US mail to-

Mary Kelly, Esq
Office of the Solicitor, USPTO, Mail Stop 8
PO Box 1450
Arlington, Va. 22313

**UNITED STATES DISTRICT COURT** FOR *EASTERN DISTRICT OF VIRGINIA*

M.R.Mikkilineni
PO Box 32110
Washington, DC 20007
      Plaintiff,
v.
                            No:09cv1412
                            Judge Brinkema

Robert Stoll, Commissioner for Patents

**Plaintiff's Motion** for *relief* under Rule 60(b)(3) and *allow* the *action* to proceed under Rule 60(d)(1) based on *new-* **evidence**

I seek *relief* from *prior*-order of this court (of April 30, 2010) under rule 60(b)(3) for *fraud* (whether intrinsic or extrinsic) or *misrepresentation* by PTO in the proceedings; and this motion filed <u>within a year</u> after the entry of the order is <u>timely</u> under rule 60(c).

Also, I request the court to grant *relief* by allowing an *action* to proceed under rule 60(d)(1)- the rule does <u>not</u> limit a court's power to entertain an independent action to *relieve* a party from an order or proceeding.

I submit a brief in support of my motion and a Complaint with *relevant*-facts (from my *original*-complaint) plus *new*-evidence on PTO's *fraud*, for this court's consideration. Today's news item in NYT is relevant to all- where the US attorney in SD of NY is busting the *drug*-gangs worldwide while the US attorney in ED of Va. is assisting PTO favor the drug-makers and bust nearly 35% of the Americans in the process...

**On April 30, 2010** (order-1), this court *"dismissed with prejudice"* my *original*-complaint based on PTO's willful *misrepresentations* of facts/law (see transcript), and said-

*"as the government has correctly pointed out,... not yet had a final agency action... patent has not finally been rejected... without a final action from the agency, .. no basis to be in this court"*.

On **December 22, 2010** (order-2), Fed. Cir. *denied* my appeal affirming order of this court on the issue- *"no basis to be in this court"* (for lack of jurisdiction); in doing so, Fed. Cir. went ahead to approve PTO's *new* rule as interpretive in the absence of jurisdiction on the issue- 'whether PTO's *new* rule is interpretive'- because, this court did not reach to that issue when it dismissed my complaint claiming lack of jurisdiction. Therefore, under our *'rule of law'*, Fed. Cir.'s opinion approving of PTO's *new* rule and the wrongful acts is *void*.

PTO is aware of its *misrepresentations* made in persuading this court (and Fed. Cir.) to dismiss my claims for lack of jurisdiction under 5 USC @551-3(c ) & (e) and 702, 706(1) & (2). Therefore, it waited until **March 23, 2011**- a day after expiry of 90-day time limit to petition USSC- and entered a *'final* rejection' of patent. In doing so, PTO freely used the *new* rule- *"purely mental process in which thoughts or human actions are changed is not considered patentable..."*- at least *five* times in rejecting evidence in my affidavit (Exb. 3.7.1) and the patent under @101 (see final-1). In conclusion PTO's *final* rejection says-

*"the examiner agrees that thoughts produce brain-neuron changes in the brain, however, these transformations are not considered an eligible transformation.."*

I may *re*-apply for patent or may appeal to the Board; but, that will not do any good until this *new* discriminatory rule is repealed or stricken by this court. Having this *new* rule in place, PTO will sit on my *re*-application for few more years, like before, and repeat its act. So, the only option I have is- come back into this court for a hearing on the merits (or go before the US Congress) and get PTO's *new* rule stricken.

Therefore, I request this court to <u>allow</u> (i) the action to proceed with discovery, and (ii) a trial by Jury on PTO's *misrepresentations* or *fraud* since this court is vested with jurisdiction under 5 USC @551-3 & 702, 706 (see brief).

I have <u>not</u> and will <u>not</u> ask this court to review PTO's *final* rejection of patent under 35 USC @101 etc. As the court is aware, jurisdiction under 5 USC @551-3 & 702, 706 in the matter, relating to PTO's *new* rule, remains in this court; whereas, the jurisdiction under 35 USC @101 etc. in the matter, relating to PTO's *final* rejection of patent, remains with Board of Patent Appeals and USDC/DC. And, there is <u>no</u> other statute or law that makes this court's jurisdiction *void* under 5 USC @551-3 & 702, 706 because of PTO's *final* rejection of patent.

Respectfully,

M.R.Mikkilineni
PO Box 32110
Washington, DC 20007

I certify that I hand delivered a copy of this pleading on March 28, 2011 to the office of US attorney ED of Va. at-

D C Barghaan, Esq.
Assist. US attorney
2100 Jamieson Ave.
Alexandria, Va. 22314

**UNITED STATES DISTRICT COURT** FOR *EASTERN DISTRICT OF VIRGINIA*

M.R.Mikkilineni
      Plaintiff,
v.                            No:09cv1412
                                   Judge Brinkema
Robert Stoll, Commissioner for Patents

**Plaintiff's *Brief*** in support of *Motion* under rule 60(b) & (d)

I submit this brief in support of my motion under rule 60(b) & (d) for relief from *prior*-order of April 30, 2010. My summary of *notarized* relevant-*facts* filed in this court on or about April 15, 2010, is true and correct; and, in my Complaint *attached*, I cite *new*-evidence from the court-transcript on PTO's *misrepresentations*.

To win or lose is <u>not</u> important to me- it is the right or wrong what each *Soul* keeps track of for use at the End. Therefore, I can <u>only</u> state the true-facts in my own word; I can <u>only</u> cite law in the words of judges, and let the court decide if true...

*First*, this court has the jurisdiction in the matter under 5 USC @531-3(c) & (e) and 702, 706(1) & (2) per the words of judges, below:

See <u>Tafas</u>, 559 F.3d 1345 (2009), where Fed. Cir. (*en banc*) said-

*"While the text of the rules sets forth a facially reasonable procedural requirement, we are mindful of the possibility that the PTO may in some cases attempt to apply the rules in a way that makes compliance essentially impossible and substantively deprives applicants of their rights. In such cases, judicial review will be available under* <u>5 USC @ 706</u>*".*

That's precisely what PTO did here- under @ 553(b)(A) made effective on Aug. 24, 2009 an Interim Guidance with a *new* rule- *"**Purely mental processes in which thoughts or human based actions are 'changed' are not considered an eligible*** *transformation*". No court in the land has <u>ever</u> made a ruling of this kind. PTO's *in-house authority* simply made this up…as if they can take '*any position under the Sun…*', and applied the *new* rule exclusively against my method *in a way that made my compliance essentially impossible and substantively deprived my right*. Therefore, in my case *judicial review is available under* 5 USC @706.

The facts show PTO's *new* rule is a change in the existing law or policy, and it is impermissibly substantive, inconsistent with law, arbitrary and capricious, incomprehensibly vague, procedurally defective. It affected my rights and obligations making my compliance essentially impossible and substantively deprived my right. Upon my timely comments and objection to the new rule based on PTO's Notice, it did <u>not</u> act to amend or *repeal* the *new* rule, and continued to misuse it against me. Thus, PTO clearly failed to take a *discrete* action it is required to take (see *relevant*-facts in the Complaint at para 10).

So, judicial review is available under 5 USC @531-3(c) & (e) and 702, 706(1) & (2).

See *Bilski*, 130 S.Ct. 3218, where Supreme Court in its recent ruling clearly rejected the notion of limitations in the existing law, and said-

"*Congress plainly contemplated that the patent laws would be given wide scope… ingenuity should receive a liberal encouragement… This court has more than once cautioned that* (lower) *courts should not read into the patent laws limitations and conditions which the legislature has not expressed. Concern about attempts to call any form of human activity a process can be met by making sure the claim meets the requirement of @101. Adopting the machine-or-transformation test as the sole test for what constitutes a process* (as opposed to just an important and useful clue) *violates these statutory principles…It is true… that a process is an act or a series of acts, performed up on the subject-matter to be transformed and reduced to a different state or thing* (and it is) *not intended to be an exhaustive or exclusive test* (because) *transformation and reduction of an article to a different state or thing is the clue to the patentability of a process claim that does not include particular machine..*"

In <u>Chrysler</u>, 441 US 281, Supreme Court said-

*"Section 10 (a) of the APA, <u>5 USC 553</u>, provides that "[a] person suffering legal wrong because of agency action, or adversely affected or aggrieved by agency action . . . , is entitled to judicial review thereof... Section 4 of the APA, specifies that an agency shall afford interested persons general notice of proposed rulemaking and an opportunity to comment before a substantive rule is promulgated... The pertinent provisions of § 10 (e) of the APA, <u>5 USC 706</u>, state that a reviewing court shall,*

*(2) hold unlawful and set aside agency action, findings, and conclusions found to be-*

*(A) arbitrary, capricious, an abuse of discretion, or otherwise not in accordance with law;*

*. . . .*

*(F) unwarranted by the facts to the extent that the facts are subject to trial de novo by the reviewing court.*

*<u>5 USC 552(a)(4)(B)</u> gives federal district courts jurisdiction to enjoin the agency from withholding agency records and to order the production of any agency records improperly withheld from the complainant.*

In <u>Norton</u>, 542 US 55, Supreme Court said-

*"The Administrative Procedure Act (APA) authorizes suit by a person suffering legal wrong because of agency action, or adversely affected or aggrieved by agency action within the meaning of a relevant statute. <u>5 USC 702</u>... Agency action is defined in <u>5 USC 551(13)</u> to include **the whole or a part of an agency rule**, order, license, sanction, relief, or the equivalent or denial thereof, or **failure to act**. The APA provides relief for a failure to act in <u>5 USC 706(1)</u>: The reviewing court shall compel agency action unlawfully withheld or unreasonably delayed".*

*"The provisions of* 5 USC 702, 704, *and* 706(1) *all insist upon an "agency action" either as* **the action complained of** *or as the action to be compelled. The definition of that term begins with a list of five categories of decisions made or outcomes implemented by an agency:* **agency rule,** *order, license, sanction, or relief.* 5 USC 551(13). *All of those categories* **involve circumscribed, discrete agency actions,** *as their definitions make clear: an agency* **statement of future effect designed to implement, interpret, or prescribe law or policy** *(rule); a final disposition in a matter other than rule making (order); a permit or other form of permission (license); a prohibition or taking of other compulsory or restrictive action (sanction); or a grant of money, assistance, license, authority, etc., or recognition of a claim, right, immunity, etc., or* **taking of other action on the** *application or* **petition of, and beneficial to, a person** *(relief).* 5 USC 551(4), (6), (8), (10), (11)".*

*"The terms following the five categories of agency action set forth in* 5 USC 551(13) *are not defined in the Administrative Procedure Act: or the equivalent or denial thereof, or failure to act. But an "equivalent thereof" must also be discrete (or it would not be equivalent), and a "denial thereof" must be the denial of a discrete listed action (and perhaps denial of a discrete equivalent). The final term in the definition set forth in* 5 USC 551(13), **"failure to act,"** *is properly understood* **as a failure to take an agency action**; *that is, a failure to take one of the agency actions (including their equivalents) earlier defined in* 551(13). *For purposes of* 5 USC 551(a), *a failure to act is not the same thing as a denial. The latter is the agency's act of saying no to a request; the former is* **simply the omission of an action without formally rejecting a request**, *for example, the failure to promulgate a rule or take some decision by a statutory deadline. The important point is that a "failure to act" is properly understood to be limited, as are the other items in* 551(13), *to* **a discrete action**".*

*"A claim under* 5 USC 706(1) *can proceed only where a plaintiff* **asserts that an agency failed to take a discrete agency action that it is required to take... Unless and until the (agency act) is amended, such actions can be set aside as contrary to law pursuant to** 5 USC 706(2)".**

And, in <u>Commonwealth</u> v. US, 2009 US Dist. LEXIS 110293, judge Friedman of USDC/DC said-

*"A party experiences actionable harm when "depriv[ed] of a procedural protection to which he is entitled" under the APA. <u>Sugar Cane Growers</u>, 289 F.3d 89. If such were not the case, "<u>sec. 553</u> would be a dead letter." If defendants have in fact violated the APA's notice-and-comment provisions, then, there is no question that the (plaintiff) will be injured by the implementation of the Interim... Rule".*

<u>Second</u>, this court can grant *relief* under rule 60(b)(3) from *prior*-order of April 30, 2010 entered as a result of PTO's *fraud* (whether intrinsic or extrinsic) or *misrepresentations* to the court. I cited *new*-evidence from the court record in my Complaint *attached*; and this motion filed <u>within a year</u> after the entry of the order is <u>timely</u> under rule 60(c). Also, the court can grant *relief* by allowing an *action* to proceed under rule 60(d)(1)- the rule does <u>not</u> limit a court's power to entertain an independent action to relieve a party from an order or proceeding.

See <u>Salazar</u>, 130 S.Ct. 1803, where the Supreme Court said-

*"Court must never ignore significant changes in the law or circumstances underlying an injunction lest the decree be turned into an instrument of wrong. A court must find prospective relief that fits the remedy to the wrong or injury..."*

In <u>Horne</u>, 129 S.Ct. 2579, Supreme Court said-

*".. courts must vigilantly enforce federal law and must not hesitate in awarding necessary relief. It takes an original judgment as a given and asks only whether a significant change in factual conditions or law renders continued enforcement of the judgment detrimental to the public interest. The rule permits relief from a judgment.. where applying it prospectively is no longer equitable.. once a party carries the burden (of showing the changed conditions), a court **abuses** its discretion when it refuses.."*

In <u>Steel</u>, 106 US at 454, Supreme Court said-

*"..if a judgment has been obtained by means (of false and perjured testimony), the remedy of the aggrieved party is to apply for a new trial, or take an appeal to a higher court; and if the testimony was accompanied with acts which prevented him from presenting to the court the merits of his case, or by which the jurisdiction of the court was imposed upon, he may also institute some direct proceeding to reach the judgment"*

*Conclusion*:

Based on the *new*-evidence cited in the Complaint and the law cited in the Brief this court has jurisdiction in the matter under APA, and FRCP rule 60(d)(1) does <u>not</u> limit this court's power to entertain an independent action to relieve from prior-order or proceeding.

Therefore, I request the court to grant relief by allowing the action to proceed expeditiously in the interest of the Public, and hold PTO's *new* rule and its misuse is unlawful being arbitrary, capricious, an abuse of discretion, contrary to constitutional right, power, privilege, and in excess of statutory jurisdiction, authority. Or enter a declaratory-order that the *new*-rule is being *applied* in this case *in a way that makes compliance essentially impossible and substantively deprives rights.*

Respectfully,

M.R.Mikkilineni
PO Box 32110
Washington, DC 20007

I certify that I hand delivered a copy of this pleading on March 28, 2011 to the office of US attorney ED of Va. at-

D C Barghaan, Esq.,
Assist. US attorney,
2100 Jamieson Ave.
Alexandria, Va. 22314

**UNITED STATES DISTRICT COURT** FOR *EASTERN DISTRICT OF VIRGINIA*

M.R.Mikkilineni
PO Box 32110
Washington, DC 20007
     Plaintiff,
v.
                          No:09cv1412
                          Judge Brinkema

Robert Stoll, Commissioner for Patents

**Plaintiff's** *request* to *re-***consider Order of** *April* 7th **that denied** *relief* under Rule 60(b)(3) & 60(d)(1)

1. On April 7th this court denied my motion for *relief* under rule 60(b)(3) for *fraud* by PTO and said-

*"plaintiff must demonstrate through clear and convincing evidence that the fraud adversely impacted 'the full and fair... presentation of its case... instead, he merely repeats the legal arguments that he already presented to this court...Moreover, the defendant's legal positions were accepted by this court and the federal circuit. Accordingly, .. Ordered that plaintiff's motion for relief under rule 60(b)(3) is denied"*.

Response: This court accepted PTO's *fraud* as the legal positions to conclude *"as the government has correctly pointed out,... not yet had a final agency action... patent has not finally been rejected... without a final action from the agency,... no basis to be in this court"* for lack of jurisdiction under 5 USC @553(e) & 706(2)...

Fed. Cir. simply rubber-stamped that *fraud* thrashing its own law in *Tafas*, 559 F.3d 1345, and made Congress law at 5 USC @553(c) & (e) and 706(2) a *'dead letter'*, like this court did in this *pro se* case. Fed. Cir. acted this way with a *non*-precedential and *un*-published opinion, and concealed its acts as if they are rooted in *'Sharia law'*- where <u>no</u> one, but a Muslim, can have jurisdiction in the court- as here a *pro se*, a *non*-Muslim, cannot have jurisdiction in our courts for a 'full and fair' hearing...

I repeated my legal arguments in my motion for relief- citing Supreme Court rulings [see *Bilski*, 130 S.Ct. 3218; *Chrysler*, 441 US 281; *Norton*, 542 US 55; *Salazar*, 130 S.Ct. 1803; *Horne*, 129 S.Ct. 2579; *Steel*, 106 US at 454] that support jurisdiction in this court under 5 USC @551-3(c)-(e) and @702, 706(1)-(2). And, I demonstrated '*clear* evidence' on PTO's *fraud* in the prior proceeding. But, this court simply refuses to review or provide for a 'full and fair' hearing to present the '*convincing* evidence', as if a *pro se* case belongs in a '*Sharia law*' court under prior rulings...despite *new*-evidence.

Here is the summary of *new*-**evidence** on PTO's *fraud or misrepresentations* (see complaint attached to my motion):

@ 12(v)  Regarding the *new* rule PTO said- "*there would be no standing for an individual...unless there was some reasonable expectation that it would be applied against them in a detrimental way*"

@ 12(vi)  In the pleadings filed PTO said- "*... Mikkilineni had an opportunity to comment on the Interim guidelines- both before and after the examiner issued an initial rejection of Mikkilineni's claims on October 27, 2009- but failed to do so undermines his current claim that the PTO deprived him of any rights under the APA*"

@ 13(i)  This court did not allow discovery or allow me present evidence; nor decide- whether the *new* rule is interpretive or substantive, or whether PTO '*failed to take a discrete action*', which it is required to take upon receiving my timely comments, to repeal the *new* rule.

@ 13(iii)  Fed. Cir. affirmed on the issue of lack of jurisdiction in a *pro se* case; and, approved PTO's *new* rule as interpretive- in the absence of jurisdiction because this court did not reach to that issue when this court claimed lack of jurisdiction. Therefore, under our '*rule of law*', Fed. Cir.'s approval of PTO's *new* rule is *void*.

@ 13(iv)  On March 23, 2011, PTO entered a *'final* rejection'
of patent. In doing so, it freely used the *new* rule *"purely mental
process in which thoughts or human actions are changed is not
considered patentable…"*, at least *five* times and admits *"the examiner
agrees that thoughts produce brain-neuron changes in the brain,
however, these transformations are not considered an eligible
transformation…"*

@ 13(v)  PTO refused to repeal the *new* rule for the second time
and disregarded my timely comments of Aug. 05, 2010 (Exb. 4.3)
in response to its latest Notice on '*Interim Bilski Guidance*'. In
*Bilski* the Supreme Court said *"concerns about attempts to call any
form of human activity a process can be met by making sure the
claim meets the requirement of @101"*; and, the Court did <u>not</u> rule
that transformation of brain-neurons thru '*mental process*' is <u>not</u>
patentable, as PTO's *new* rule says without any basis.

In fact, even under '*Sharia law*' in a *pro se* case, Fed. Cir. admits
that PTO's notice in <u>*Animal*</u>, 932 F.2d at 920 *"mirrored the Supreme
Court's holding in <u>Diamond</u>, 447 US at 309"*- therefore, that notice
was interpretive. Whereas, in this *pro se* case evidence shows PTO's
repeated use of a *new* rule that did <u>not</u> *"mirror"* the Supreme Court's
holding in <u>*Bilski*</u>, 130 S.Ct. 3218, or any other court in the land-
besides the '*Sharia law*' courts…

@ 13(vi)  Thus, PTO continued to discriminate my 'process' for
nearly 5-years, *first* through the '*in-house authority*', then, put into
effect a *new* rule- that made my compliance essentially impossible,
and substantively deprived my rights under 5 USC @ 551-3(c) & (e)
and 702, 706(1) & (2).

2.  On April 7th this court refused to grant *relief* by allowing an *action*
to proceed under rule 60(d)(1) and said (at note 1)-

*"Other powers to grant relief. This rule does not limit a court's power
to entertain an independent action to relieve a party from a.. order..
This rule does not provide a separate basis for relief.. therefore, the
court considers this motion only under FRCP 60(b)"*.

<u>Response</u>: Certainly, rule 60(d)(1) does <u>not</u> limit this court's power to entertain an independent action based on *new*-evidence, and under the circumstances where PTO has continued doing wrongful acts using the *new* rule as a substantive rule and entered a final rejection of patent. Even if the courts- in the prior proceeding- *mis*took PTO's real intent in creating that *new* rule, it should be clear, at least now- that the wrongful acts of PTO are the cause for suffering of nearly 35% of our-fellow citizens with 'sleep' related problems and get addicted to the drugs… When the US attorney/SD of NY (and the judges) are busting the drug-gangs worldwide, the US attorney/ED of Va. (and the judges) are assisting PTO push drugs upon nearly 35% of our-fellow citizens…

The decision of this court <u>not</u> to assert power under rule 60(d)(1) with a pretext the rule *"does not provide a separate basis for relief"*, must be a continued act to use *'Sharia law'* knowing the appeal court rubber stamps the order in a pro se case. And, it does not matter how it impacts upon fellow citizens- who are believers in *'Father'* and *'Holy ghost'*, like I am…

Respectfully,

M.R.Mikkilineni
PO Box 32110
Washington, DC 20007

I certify that I hand delivered a copy of this pleading on April 18, 2011 to the office of US attorney ED of Va. at-
D C Barghaan, Esq.,
Assist. US attorney,
2100 Jamieson Ave.
Alexandria, Va. 22314

# UNITED STATES COURT OF APPEALS FOR THE FEDERAL Cir.

## No. 2011-1389

M.R.Mikkilineni
        Plaintiff-Appellant,
v.

Robert Stoll, Commissioner of Patents,
        Defendant-Appellee.

Appeal from the United States District Court for the Eastern District of Virginia, Case No. 09-cv-1412, Judge Leonie M. Brinkema.

*Informal Brief of Appellant* (Appendix attached)

On this date, June 7, 2011, I file one original and three copies of *signed* 2-page informal brief with 11-extra sheets answering questions 1-6 (plus orders for review 3 pages; proposed complaint w/exhibits 28 pages; docket entries 4 pages)- total 48 pages- for review by the panel.

**1.** Factual background:

Five years ago, upon perfecting the "process" to fall asleep *instantly*, I applied for a patent. The process flips off the 'light-switch' in the brain-stem, and activates '*master clock*' in the brain for a sleep-cycle.

The process *transforms specific-neurons* in the brain into a different state to make them active, and produces melatonin and serotonin to activate the '*master clock*' for a sleep-cycle. Thus, the process tunes brain off intrusive thoughts streaming into the mind due to anxiety, anger, depression or mental-disorder(s).

The brain with 2-hemispheres communicates with each other- one thought at a time; any interference in the brain caused by 2 or more thoughts coming into the mind at the same instant creates havoc with motor responses, and the 2-hemispheres stop communicating- a split brain. That split brain causes light switch flip and activates the *master-clock* to make the brain fall asleep- thus, helps cure depression or mental-disorder(s). A recent study at Harvard Medical School and University of California concludes-

*"...a lack of sleep causes the brain's emotional centers to dramatically overreact...(with) psychiatric disorders... (and) fractures the brain mechanisms that regulate key aspects of mental health... and, sleep appears to restore emotional brain's circuits...."*

Prescription sleeping-pills can cause strange and potentially dangerous side effects. And, at this stage, science is trying to find a way to implant a new *'gene'* or light switch in the brain to treat mental-disorder(s), and/or control sleep-wake state of the brain with a flip of the light switch; but, science is unable to locate or repair the light switch that exist in the brain-stem. Whereas, my process repairs the existing light switch in the brain and makes it work <u>without</u> using an implant or drug.

I filed for a patent, because if I put the process into practice without a patent protection the sleeping-pill makers could start a parallel organization to drive me out, and keep making money selling pills...

In May 2007, patent attorney Swift and I met supervisor-examiner Pezzuto; his interview summary states *"there is no agreement as the rejection under 35 USC 101 and the examiner will discuss this with in-house authorities"*

Later, Mr.Pezzuto indicated likelihood of granting patent; but, in October 2007, a Jr. examiner (working for Pezzuto) sent a **final** rejection per the *dictates* of *in-house authority*.

In December 2007, I filed for patent 2nd time (CiP1); PTO sent my application for review by a new-examiner. In August 2008, I met examiner Gilbert and explained- how any person interested in learning the skill can be trained for a beneficial use of my method. Mr.Gilbert understood and his interview summary states:

*"Mr.Mikkilineni explained that his method was not concentrating on a scene with two elements of an image at the same time, but, keep two separate elements as two separate thoughts,* (and) *bring them into the mind at the same time"*.

I also made it clear that a specification or a book can't teach some-one ride a bike or an MD-trainee perform brain-Surgery before learning the art in a teaching school- if books can enable an ordinary skilled to learn on his/her own, there is no need for a teaching school- like the one I intend to start and teach the method.

In June 2008, examiner sent claim rejections (non-final) under 35 USC @101, 112.

In September 2008, I had a telephone interview with supervisor-examiner Marmor, and his summary says:

*"Applicant explained... and suggested a sleep study be conducted to address the rejections... examiner explained that the sleep study would likely **not be useful**... that the pending method claims involve **merely mental steps** and are unpatentable and **nonstatutory**. A patent eligible process under 35 USC 101 must be tied to another statutory class, such as a particular apparatus, or **transform** underlying subject matter or material"*.

My method is not *"merely mental steps"*; PTO's *in-house authority* mislabeled to *kill* it.

In October 2008, patent attorney Swift filed CiP2, a new application (at No.12/259,285).

In September 2009, I discovered an article published in Washington Post titled '*Meditation Gives Brain a Charge...*'- a study conducted at U. of Wisconsin with the help of **Dalai Lama** (the study-results were published by **National Academy of Sciences**). I forwarded that article to the examiner.

In October 2009, examiner sent claim *rejection* (non-final) under 35 USC @101, 112.

In October 2009, Mr.Swift and I met examiner Gilbert, and supervisor-examiner Marmor:

Mr.Marmor gave me a copy of a **new 'guidance' dated August 24, 2009**, and pointing to a sentence that *"Purely mental processes in which thoughts or human based actions are 'changed' are not considered an eligible transformation"*, informed me of his **inability to accept my method for a patent under that *new* rule.**

In October 2009, well before the deadline date of November 9, 2009, I sent a petition to Commissioner Stoll (Exb. 3.6) for repeal of that *new* rule. PTO did not act and kept the *new* rule in place after having discriminated my method since 2006 in favor of pill makers; thus, violated my right to due process under 5 USCS § 553(c) & (e).

PTO's failure is arbitrary, capricious, and an abuse of discretion or otherwise not in accordance with law; or contrary to constitutional right, power, privilege, or immunity; or in excess of statutory jurisdiction, authority or limitations; and without observance of procedure required by law- under @ 706(2)(A), (B), (C), (D). Therefore, in December 2009, I filed a complaint in USDC/ED of Va. at No.09cv1412.

On April 30, 2010, trial court- *"dismissed with prejudice"* my complaint- using PTO's willful *misrepresentations* of facts/law said-

*"as the government has correctly pointed out,… not yet had a final agency action… patent has not finally been rejected… without a final action from the agency, .. no basis to be in this court".*

On December 22, 2010, Fed. Cir. *denied* my appeal and affirmed the order of trial court on the issue- *"no basis to be in this court"* (for lack of jurisdiction). Fed. Cir., on its own, approved PTO's guideline (including the *new* rule) as 'interpretive' in the <u>absence of jurisdiction</u> to decide on an issue- 'whether the *new* rule is interpretive'; because, the trial court did <u>not</u> reach to that issue when it dismissed the complaint for lack of jurisdiction under 5 USC @553, 706.

**2.** *New* evidence:

PTO is aware of its *misrepresentations* made to the courts in persuading the courts to dismiss my claims for lack of jurisdiction under 5 USC @553(c ) & (e) and 702, 706(2). So, PTO waited until March 23, 2011, or until the 90-day time to petition USSC had expired, before entering a '**final** rejection' of patent (see Final-1). In doing so, PTO has freely used the *new* rule- "*purely mental process in which thoughts or human actions are changed is not considered patentable…*"- at least **five** times in rejecting evidence in my affidavit (Exb.3.7.1) and the patent under @101. In conclusion, PTO said:

"*the examiner agrees that thoughts produce brain-neuron changes in the brain, however, these transformations are not considered an eligible transformation.*"

Thus, PTO applied it's so called '*interpretive*' rule as a '*substantive*' rule against my method in its **final** rejection of patent. Even if I decide to *re*-apply for a patent 3rd time (CiP3), it will <u>not</u> do any good until this *new* substantive rule is repealed or stricken. Having this *new* rule in place, PTO will sit on my application for few more years, like before, and repeat its act. So, the <u>only</u> option I have is to file a motion for relief from prior-order under rule 60(b) & (d) [or go before the US Congress] to get the *new* rule stricken.

**3.** *Material* facts including ***new***-evidence on PTO's *fraud*:

On March 28, 2011, within a year from the date of original-dismissal, I filed a rule 60(b)(3) & (d)(1) motion in the trial-court with a request to <u>allow</u> (i) the action to proceed with discovery, and (ii) a trial by Jury on PTO's *fraud*- as the court is vested with jurisdiction under 5 USC @551-3 & 702, 706 (see complaint plus exhibits attached).

I have <u>not</u> asked the court to review PTO's **final** rejection of patent under 35 USC @101.

For PTO's *fraud* upon the courts, see the summary below (from transcript of 04/30/2010).

(i) PTO (on p.3, L24-5): *"when the examiner enters final rejections,… he'll have the ability to appeal at that time"*.

PTO knew *final* rejection and appeal is <u>not</u> the issue in my claim under 5 USC @553(c) & (e) and 706- I asserted claim for denial of my rights under the *new* rule, and requested the court to decide whether PTO's *new*-rule is substantive.

(ii) PTO (on p.4, L23-4): *"PTO made very clear that because it is an interpretive rule, it's not substantive rule making,"*.

PTO knew under the guise of interpretive rules it included this *new* rule, a *substantive* rule with an intent to deprive my rights under 5 USC @531-3(c) & (e) and 702, 706(1) & (2), and upon my timely comments it did <u>not</u> repeal the *new* rule.

(iii) PTO (on p.5, L19-25): *"Fed. Cir. has said very clearly that it has the authority to tell the PTO that its interpretive guidance is wrong… on the merits, correct. That when it receives an appeal from the Patent Board of a rejection of a particular patent application from an applicant like Mikkilineni,…"*.

PTO knew the court has jurisdiction under 5 USC @553(c) & (e) and 706 to tell the PTO its *new* rule is wrong, and Mikkilineni need not wait for Patent Board rejection of appeal under 35 USC @101 etc. since these two statutes are different.

(iv) PTO (on p.7, L1-3): *"there would be no standing for an individual…unless there was some reasonable expectation that it would be applied against them in a detrimental way,"*.

PTO knew it applied the *new* rule against me in a detrimental way for nearly 5 years.

(v) PTO's pleadings (filed in the courts) said "... *Mikkilineni had an opportunity to comment on the Interim guidelines- both before and after the examiner issued an initial rejection of Mikkilineni's claims on October 27, 2009- but failed to do so undermines his current claim that the PTO deprived him of any rights under the APA*".

PTO knew I timely filed comments (see Exb.3.6 & 4.3) in response to the Notices; and PTO did not act to repeal the *new* rule.

Using PTO's willful *misrepresentations*, on 4/30/2010, trial-court *"dismissed with prejudice"* my Complaint, and did not allow discovery or present evidence. The court did not decide- whether the *new* rule is interpretive or substantive, and bypassed the issue- whether PTO has '*failed to take a discrete action*' which it is required to take upon receiving my timely comments or repeal the *new* rule.

(vi) On 12/22/2010, Fed. Cir. affirmed trial-court's decision that *"no basis to be in this court"* (for lack of jurisdiction), and approved PTO's *new* rule as interpretive. It did so, in the absence of jurisdiction on 'whether PTO's *new* rule is interpretive' because, trial-court did not reach to that issue when it dismissed my complaint for lack of jurisdiction. So, under our '*rule of law*', Fed. Cir.'s opinion approving of PTO's *new* rule is *void*.

(vii) PTO, on March 23, 2011- one day after expiry of 90-day time to petition USSC- entered a '**final** rejection' of patent. In doing so, PTO freely used the *new* rule- *"purely mental process in which thoughts or human actions are changed is not considered patentable..."*- at least **five** times to reject evidence in my affidavit (Exb. 3.7.1) and patent under @101 (**final**-1); and, in conclusion, PTO said:

*"the examiner agrees that thoughts produce brain-neuron changes in the brain, however, these transformations are not considered an eligible transformation.."*

(viii)  On 8/05/2010, I filed timely comments second time (Exb. 4.3), in response to PTO's subsequent-Notice on '*Interim Bilski Guidance*'. PTO, again, refused to repeal the *new* rule.

In *Bilski* the Supreme Court said- "*concerns about attempts to call any form of human activity a process can be met by making sure the claim meets the requirement of @101*"- and, the Court did <u>not</u> rule that transformation of brain-neurons thru '*mental process*' is <u>not</u> patentable as PTO's *new* rule says…

(ix)  Thus, PTO continued to discriminate my process for nearly 5-years, *first* through the '*in-house authority*', then, put into effect a *new* rule to make my compliance essentially impossible, and substantively deprived my rights under 5 USC @ 551-3(c) & (e) and 702, 706(1) & (2).

**4.**  <u>Issue(s) for *Review* by Fed.Cir.</u>:

On 4/07/2011, trial-court denied my motion for *relief* under rule 60(b) (3) for *fraud* by PTO and said-

"*plaintiff must demonstrate through clear and convincing evidence that the fraud adversely impacted 'the full and fair… presentation of its case…Moreover, the defendant's legal positions were accepted by this court and the federal circuit. Accordingly, .. Ordered that plaintiff's motion for relief under rule 60(b)(3) is denied*".

**Issue 1**:  Did the Courts *err*?

Yes. Courts have *erred* in accepting PTO's *fraud* as the '*legal positions*', and made a *new*-law from the bench in a *pro se* case thrashing the law of Congress at 5 USC @553(c) (e) & 706(2)… as a "*dead letter*".

*First*, court-record shows (see transcript of 4/30/2010) court did <u>not</u> allow discovery nor allow presentation of evidence at the hearing. And, it refused to take jurisdiction in the matter under a pretext "*as the government has correctly pointed out, ... patent has not finally been rejected... without a final action from the agency, ... no basis to be in this court"*.

Fed. Cir. affirmed that decision in a non-precedential un-published opinion as if '*Sharia law*' is applicable in a *pro se* case- where <u>no</u> one, but a Muslim, can have rights; here, a *pro se*, a *non*-Muslim, cannot have right for a 'full and fair' hearing.

Obviously, <u>*Tafas*</u>, 559 F.3d 1345, is <u>not</u> applicable to a *pro se* case as it only applies to the rights of non *pro se* where the Fed. Cir. said:

*"While the text of the rules sets forth a facially reasonable procedural requirement, we are mindful of the possibility that the PTO may in some cases attempt to apply the rules in a way that makes compliance essentially impossible and substantively deprives applicants of their rights. In such cases, judicial review will be available under* <u>5 USC @ 706</u>".

*Second*, although the trial-court refused to decide 'whether PTO's *new* rule is interpretive', Fed. Cir. went ahead to approve PTO's guidance (including that one *new* substantive rule) as interpretive- in the absence of jurisdiction- and said:
*"our decision in* <u>Animal</u>... *is almost directly on point"*, because PTO's notice in <u>Animal</u>... *"mirrored the Supreme Court's holding in* <u>Diamond</u>...(so) *this court rejected th*(at) *plaintiff's argument, finding that the PTO notice was interpretive rather than substantive"*.

There it made sense because in <u>Animal</u> PTO's notice simply "*mirrored*" the law of the highest court in the land; however, it is not clear how <u>Animal</u> "*is almost directly on point"* in my case. Here, there is <u>no</u> such law to *mirror* or enable PTO making a *new* substantive rule at will to justify discrimination of my method since 2006. It is simple, and <u>not</u> hard to see the difference between <u>Animal</u>... and my present case.

Although under our '*rule of law*', Fed. Cir.'s approval of a *new* rule is *void*, PTO in its latest pleading (filed on 4/06/2011), again, makes false or twisted 'legal positions', as usual-

(i) "*..court continues to lack jurisdiction over plaintiff's attempt* (under rule 60b) *to have court review the substantive doctrine that has been applied by examiner to his patent application*"

It is not clear what is meant by "*substantive doctrine.. applied by examiner*" to my application. If it means the "*examiner agrees that thoughts produce brain-neuron changes in the brain* (but) *these transformations are not considered an eligible transformation*" under PTO's *new* rule (see **3**vii)- that's <u>not</u> the law of Congress, nor the law of a court; and PTO simply made that up, on its own, in the absence of authority.

(ii) "*..Fed Cir. holding that* (PTO) *guidance is an interpretive rule exempt from APA's notice and comment requirements applies with equal force.. to which the Fed Cir. pointed in holding that the earlier guidance document was 'interpretive' and thus APA exempt*"

Using Fed Cir.'s <u>void</u> order on the guidance, PTO justifies its use of a *substantive* rule against my method here. The trial-court did <u>not</u> take evidence, nor rule whether or not that <u>one</u> *new*-rule in earlier guidance was interpretive; and, Fed Cir. knew it had <u>no</u>-jurisdiction to decide on that <u>one</u> *new*-rule. Therefore, panel muddled through that issue using words such as- <u>Animal</u> *mirrored* <u>Diamond</u>, guidance is interpretive and exempt from APA etc…

PTO lawyers and the panel knew I did <u>not</u> ask the courts to decide whether the guidance is interpretive; instead, I asked the courts to decide whether that <u>one</u> *new*-rule was substantive and, whether that <u>one</u> *new*-rule made my compliance essentially impossible, and substantively deprived my rights under 5 USC @ 551-3(c) & (e) and 702, 706(1) & (2).

The lawyers, judge and the panel understood the issue clearly; therefore, decided to apply '*Sharia law*' to this pro se, like the Islamists do to a *non*-Muslim all the time.

On 4/07/2011, judge denied relief under rule 60(b)(3) and said:

*"plaintiff must demonstrate through clear and convincing evidence that the fraud adversely impacted 'the full and fair… presentation of its case…"*

Using PTO's pleading of 4/06/2011, trial-court entered an order on 4/07/2011 removing a hearing set for 4/08/2011; thus, the court did not allow me to *"demonstrate through clear and convincing evidence that the fraud adversely impacted 'the full and fair… presentation of its case…".* Evidently, the court decided not to review the evidence I presented in my complaint attached, either, such as- PTO, on March 23, 2011, entered a '**final** rejection' of patent using the *new* rule- *"purely mental process in which thoughts or human actions are changed is not considered patentable…"*- at least **five** times to reject patent under @101 (see **3**vii). This is a *clear and convincing evidence of fraud* by PTO or its agents upon the courts who obtained orders persuading the court (i) it lacked jurisdiction because there was no **final**-rejection of patent, and (ii) the *new*-rule was interpretive. Then, soon thereafter, decided to use the *new*-rule as a *substantive* rule to enter a **final**-rejection of patent.

On 4/07/2011, judge did not consider to allow an independent action under rule 60(d)(1) and said (see order, at note 1):

*"FRCP 60(d)(1) states: other powers to grant relief. This rule does not limit a court's power to entertain an independent action to relieve a party from judgment, order, or proceeding. This rule does not provide a separate basis for relief from final judgment"*

Certainly, rule 60(d)(1) does not limit court's power to entertain an independent action based on *new*-evidence and given the circumstances where PTO has continued doing the wrongful acts using the *new* rule as a *substantive* rule to enter a **final** rejection of patent. Even if one assumes that the courts, in the prior proceeding, have *mis*took PTO's real intent in creating that *new* rule, it should be clear, at least, now that the wrongful acts are the cause of suffering for nearly 35% of our-fellow citizens with 'sleep' related problems or getting addicted to drugs.

The US attorney/SD of NY and the judges are busting the drug-gangs worldwide. The US attorney/ED of Va., PTO lawyers and the judges here help push drugs upon nearly 35% of our-fellow citizens… with a decision <u>not</u> to assert power under rule 60(d)(1) under a pretext that the rule "*does not provide a separate basis for relief*"- a continued use of '*Sharia law*' against this *pro se*.

**5.** <u>*Argument*</u>:

The evidence cited above demonstrates *clear* and *convincing* evidence on PTO's *fraud* upon the courts in prior proceeding. So, the court has jurisdiction under 5 USC @531-3(c) & (e) and 702, 706(1) & (2) to review the evidence, and grant relief under rule 60(b)(3) or allow an independent action under rule 60(d)(1).

See Supreme Court rulings in <u>*Bilski*</u>, 130 S.Ct. 3218; <u>*Chrysler*</u>, 441 US 281; <u>*Norton*</u>, 542 US 55; <u>*Salazar*</u>, 130 S.Ct. 1803; <u>*Horne*</u>, 129 S.Ct. 2579; <u>*Steel*</u>, 106 US at 454.

In <u>*Bilski*</u>, 130 S.Ct. 3218, the Court clearly rejected the notion of limitations in the existing law @101, and said-

"*Congress plainly contemplated that the patent laws would be given wide scope… ingenuity should receive a liberal encouragement… This court has more than once cautioned that* (lower) *courts should not read into the patent laws limitations and conditions which the legislature has not expressed. Concern about attempts to call any form of human activity a process can be met by making sure the claim meets the requirement of @101. Adopting the machine-or-transformation test as the sole test for what constitutes a process* (as opposed to just an important and useful clue) *violates these statutory principles…It is true… that a process is an act or a series of acts,*

*performed up on the subject-matter to be transformed and reduced to
a different state or thing* (and it is) *not intended to be an exhaustive
or exclusive test* (because) *transformation and reduction of an article
to a different state or thing is the clue to the patentability of a process
claim that does not include particular machine.."*

In <u>Chrysler</u>, 441 US 281, the Court said-

*"Section 10 (a) of the APA, <u>5 USC 553</u>, provides that "[a] person
suffering legal wrong because of agency action, or adversely affected
or aggrieved by agency action . . . , is entitled to judicial review
thereof... Section 4 of the APA, specifies that an agency shall afford
interested persons general notice of proposed rulemaking and an
opportunity to comment before a substantive rule is promulgated...
The pertinent provisions of § 10 (e) of the APA, <u>5 USC 706</u>, state that
a reviewing court shall,*

*(2) hold unlawful and set aside agency action, findings, and
conclusions found to be-*

*(A) arbitrary, capricious, an abuse of discretion, or otherwise not in
accordance with law;*

. . . .

*(F) unwarranted by the facts to the extent that the facts are subject to
trial de novo by the reviewing court.*

<u>5 USC 552(a)(4)(B)</u> *gives federal district courts jurisdiction to
enjoin the agency from withholding agency records and to order
the production of any agency records improperly withheld from the
complainant.*

In <u>Norton</u>, 542 US 55, the Court said-

*"The Administrative Procedure Act (APA) authorizes suit by a person
suffering legal wrong because of agency action, or adversely affected
or aggrieved by agency action within the meaning of a relevant*

statute. 5 USC 702... *Agency action is defined in* 5 USC 551(13) *to include **the whole or a part of an agency rule**, order, license, sanction, relief, or the equivalent or denial thereof, or **failure to act**. The APA provides relief for a failure to act in* 5 USC 706(1): *The reviewing court shall compel agency action unlawfully withheld or unreasonably delayed".*

"*The provisions of* 5 USC 702, 704, *and* 706(1) *all insist upon an "agency action" either as **the action complained of** or as the action to be compelled. The definition of that term begins with a list of five categories of decisions made or outcomes implemented by an agency: **agency rule,** order, license, sanction, or relief.* 5 USC 551(13). *All of those categories **involve circumscribed, discrete agency actionsstatement of future effect designed to implement, interpret, or prescribe law or policy** (rule); a final disposition in a matter other than rule making (order); a permit or other form of permission (license); a prohibition or taking of other compulsory or restrictive action (sanction); or a grant of money, assistance, license, authority, etc., or recognition of a claim, right, immunity, etc., or **taking of other action on the** application or **petition of, and beneficial to, a person** (relief).* 5 USC 551(4), (6), (8), (10), (11)".

"*The terms following the five categories of agency action set forth in* 5 USC 551(13) *are not defined in the Administrative Procedure Act: or the equivalent or denial thereof, or failure to act. But an "equivalent thereof" must also be discrete (or it would not be equivalent), and a "denial thereof" must be the denial of a discrete listed action (and perhaps denial of a discrete equivalent). The final term in the definition set forth in* 5 USC 551(13), "**failure to act,**" *is properly understood **as a failure to take an agency action**; that is, a failure to take one of the agency actions (including their equivalents) earlier defined in* 551(13). *For purposes of* 5 USC 551(a), *a failure to act is not the same thing as a denial. The latter is the agency's act of saying no to a request; the former is **simply the omission of an action without formally rejecting a request**, for example, the failure to promulgate a rule or take some decision by a statutory deadline. The important point is that a "failure to act" is properly understood to be limited, as are the other items in* 551(13), *to **a discrete action**".*

*"A claim under 5 USC 706(1) can proceed only where a plaintiff **asserts that an agency failed to take a discrete agency action that it is required to take… Unless and until the (agency act) is amended, such actions can be set aside as contrary to law pursuant to 5 USC 706(2)**".*

In Commonwealth v. US, 2009 US Dist. LEXIS 110293, judge Friedman of USDC/DC said-

*"A party experiences actionable harm when "depriv[ed] of a procedural protection to which he is entitled" under the APA. Sugar Cane Growers, 289 F.3d 89. If such were not the case, "sec. 553 would be a dead letter." If defendants have in fact violated the APA's notice-and-comment provisions, then, there is no question that the (plaintiff) will be injured by the implementation of the Interim… Rule".*

The court can grant *relief* under rule 60(b)(3) from *prior*-orders entered as a result of PTO's *fraud* (whether intrinsic or extrinsic) or *misrepresentations* to the court; and, the motion filed within a year after the entry of the order was timely under rule 60(c). On the basis of *new*-evidence alleged in the complaint *attached* the court can grant *relief* by allowing an *action* to proceed under rule 60(d)(1)- the rule does not limit a court's power to entertain an independent action to relieve a party from an order or proceeding.

See Salazar, 130 S.Ct. 1803, where the Supreme Court said-

*"Court must never ignore significant changes in the law or circumstances underlying an injunction lest the decree be turned into an instrument of wrong. A court must find prospective relief that fits the remedy to the wrong or injury…"*

In Horne, 129 S.Ct. 2579, Supreme Court said-

*".. courts must vigilantly enforce federal law and must not hesitate in awarding necessary relief. It takes an original judgment as a given and asks only whether a significant change in factual conditions or law renders continued enforcement of the judgment detrimental to*

*the public interest. The rule permits relief from a judgment.. where applying it prospectively is no longer equitable.. once a party carries the burden* (of showing the changed conditions), *a court **abuses** its discretion when it refuses.."*

In <u>Steel</u>, 106 US at 454, Supreme Court said-

*"..if a judgment has been obtained by means (of false and perjured testimony), the remedy of the aggrieved party is to apply for a new trial, or take an appeal to a higher court; and if the testimony was accompanied with acts which prevented him from presenting to the court the merits of his case, or by which the jurisdiction of the court was imposed upon, he may also institute some direct proceeding to reach the judgment"*

**6**. *Action* Fed.Cir. *can Take*:

I request the panel to review the evidence in the record and the law cited and remand the case to the trial-court to grant relief under rule 60(b)(1) and/or allow an independent action to proceed under rule 60(d)(1).

Respectfully,

M.R.Mikkilineni
PO Box 32110
Washington, DC 20007

Certificate of Service

I certify that I served a copy of this pleading on June 7, 2011 by hand-delivering at the office of Solicitor at the address below:
Mary Kelly, Esq
Office of the Solicitor, USPTO
Madison W, 08C43: 600 Dulany St.
Alexandria, Va. 22313

**UNITED STATES COURT OF APPEALS** FOR THE FEDERAL Cir.

**No. 2011-1389**

M.R.Mikkilineni
        Plaintiff-Appellant,
v.

Robert Stoll, Commissioner of Patents,
        Defendant-Appellee.

Appeal from the United States District Court for the Eastern District of Virginia, Case No. 09-cv-1412, Judge Leonie M. Brinkema.

*__Reply__ of Appellant* to the __Brief__ of Appellee

Please allow me to get straight to the issue involved in the present appeal, and on PTO's fraud and/or continued misrepresentations in its brief filed on 07/18/2011:

Issue: Whether 5 USC @553 (c)&(e), 702 & 706 provide jurisdiction in the district court/ED of Va. based on the **new**-evidence that PTO has used the *new*-rule as a *substantive* rule in March 2010 and made my compliance impossible depriving my rights, or that statute is still a dead-letter in my case under 35 USC @101 & 112 ?

The law of this court in Tafas, 559 F.3d 1345 (2009) provides jurisdiction under 5 USC @706 when PTO attempts to apply a new-rule *"in a way that makes compliance essentially impossible and substantively deprives applicants of their rights"*. See Norton, 542 US 55.

So, the statute 5 USC @553, 702, 706 is not a dead letter under 35 USC @101, 112; but, PTO's misrepresentations make it dead in a *pro se* case and the courts have agreed to in the first round. In the second round, this court should at least ask:

. Why the district court, in this *pro se* case, adopted *"no basis to be in this court"* (A47, L.24)] accepting PTO's misrepresentations that an article III court could review (A45 L.8-15) *"interpretive guidance on the merits"* (PTO brief on p.11) only *"when it receives an appeal from the patent Board of a rejection of a patent application from Mikkilineni"*(A45).

. Why the same court in March 2011 declares *"Plaintiff fails to meet the clear and convincing evidence standard"* (A2) having clear and convincing evidence in the record- the entry of PTO's final rejection misusing a new-substantive rule *"purely mental process in which thoughts or human actions are changed is not considered patentable eligible subject matter"* (A27-9) against this *pro se*.

Now, this court should look at PTO's continued willful misrepresentations in its brief filed in this court on 07/18/2011:

See PTO's Rebuttal on Assertion #6 (p.13-15):

(1) "Mikkilineni's alleged 'timely comments' to the.. guidelines were sent either too late or to the wrong address…Request provided that public comments should be sent via email to AB98,Comments@ uspto.gov", and must be received on or before November 9, 2009 to be considered. See A82." (p.13)

*Reply*: On **October 28, 2009** (13-days prior to the dead line date of November 9, 2009), I emailed my comments to the examiner and **faxed to PTO at 571 273 0125** (see Exb. 3.6, A37); and, PTO's Notice (A82) said *"Comments may also be submitted by facsimile to 571 273 0125"*. This shows PTO continues to make willful misrepresentations, even **now**- because that's the culture.

(2) "The second comment, which Mikkilineni labels Exb. 4.3 (A19), was addressed to Bilski_Guidance@uspto.gov -*i.e.*, the wrong address- and sent on August 5, 2010- i.e., well after the period for response had lapse…" (p.14)

*Reply*:  PTO conveniently omitted to attach a copy of its own 'Notice' in the Federal Register/ Vol. 75, No. 143/ July 27, 2010 (see p.43922 of Exb.4.1 attached) which said *"To be ensured of consideration, written comments must be received on or before **September 27, 2010** ... Comments .. should be sent by **electronic mail message** over the Internet to **Bilski_Guidance@uspto.gov**"*

As seen in Exb. 4.3 (A39), on **August 05, 2010** (52-days prior to the deadline date of September 27, 2010), I sent my comments in an **email to Bilski_Guidance@uspto.gov** That shows PTO made *knowingly false-statements* in its brief, and claims that PTO *"could not have engaged in fraud... where Mikkilineni's own evidence shows that he did not timely and properly file comments to the Guidelines"*- which is another *false* statement on top of all willful deceit in the matter during the past 5 years.

(3)  "To the extent that Mikkilineni seeks to raise new arguments in his brief to this court (at 5-6, vi-ix), he has waived these arguments by failing to present them to the district court in the first instance" (p.15)

*Reply*:  No, I did not raise any new issues in my brief filed in this court on June 7, 2011; the issues on p.5-6 at vi-ix are the same I raised in the district court at item 13 in my Complaint attached to my Motion for relief of March 28, 2011 (see A11 & A19-20).

See PTO's Rebuttal on Assertion #1, 2 & 3 (p.9-11):

(4)  "PTO correctly informed the district court that Mikkilineni can appeal the final rejection of his patent claims, along with any laws and reasoning... for the rejection, to the Board; and...to a district court (under 35 USC...)..."

*Reply*: That is a willful misrepresentation because PTO knew I made the claims under 5 USC@553, 706, not under 35 USC.

(5)  "..the district court...considered whether the Interim Guidelines are substantive rulemaking. See A45 L.23 to A46 L.15..."

*Reply*: That is a willful misrepresentation. The district court did not consider nor decide whether the Guideline or the new-rule is interpretive. See A45-A46.

(6) "there is no requirement that PTO repeal rulemaking…PTO cannot be said to have engaged in fraud… simply because the courts have agreed (with PTO)…"

*Reply*:  PTO knew my claim is under 5 USC @553, 706, and knowingly invoked 35 USC, a statute not applicable to my pending claim. Misrepresenting a final rejection of patent is required to have jurisdiction in an article III court, PTO made the district court to dismiss my claims for lack of jurisdiction. PTO's claim that *"there is no requirement"* to repeal the new substantive rule under 5 USC @553(e) is an issue to be decided by a court, if the statute is not a dead letter in a *pro se* case..

See PTO's Rebuttal on Assertion #4 & 5 (p.12):

(7) "Both the district court and this court have issued decisions holding that a district court in ED of Va. lacks the authority in an APA suit to review the merits of PTO interpretive guidance where there has been no final agency action. See A45… Because there is no error in the PTO's statements, there can be no fraud…" (p.12)

*Reply*:  The issue, **then** and **now**, is- whether the statute 5 USC @553, 702, 706 is a dead letter in this *pro se* case where PTO has applied its new-rule in such a way "that made my compliance essentially impossible and substantively deprived my rights". See Tafas, 559 F.3d 1345 (2009) and Norton, 542 US 55. As a result of PTO's, **then**, willful misrepresentations on the issue of jurisdiction the district court declared 'no jurisdiction' under 5 USC @553, 706 and the Fed. Cir. affirmed it; thus, PTO's, **then**, wrongful acts is a fraud upon the courts, which denied due process and prevented a full and fair hearing to present my case; and, **now**, PTO is repeating the same act.

(8) "…PTO was responding to (the judge) that a patent applicant lacks standing to challenge the merits of PTO guidance unless the applicant's claims have been finally rejected…" (p.12)

A133

*Reply*: Here, PTO admits to have persuaded the judge that I had no standing to make claims under 5 USC @553, 706. The judge and PTO talk *"to the extent that an applicant exercises that avenue of article III review..."* (A46 L13) with respect to the statute 35 USC ..., is not part of my present-claim under 5 USC @553, 706. Therefore, that entire hearing held on 04/30/2010 has been used by PTO to deceive the court talking about an unrelated statute and misled the judge to deny a full and fair hearing and prevented me from presenting evidence on my claims under 5 USC @553, 706.

PTO, in its brief (p.13) says *"PTO is not required to repeal rulemaking or change its practice in view of any one public comment, as Mikkilineni suggests"*.

As the record shows, since Mikkilineni's rights are the ONLY ones that particular *new*-rule has adversely effected and no one-else, that substantive rule should be repealed or stricken under 5 USC @553(e) unless PTO can show evidence that that has been its practice to make new substantive rule, selectively, from time to time and reject patents. Then, it can make an interesting Book for the People to read find how the officials are doing the 'duty' for the People.

Conclusion:

Based on the stated facts and law in my brief filed on June 7, 2011, I request this court to vacate the prior orders and remand the case into the district court for discovery in the matter and further proceedings in the interest of justice...

Respectfully,
M.R.Mikkilineni, PO Box 32110, Washington, DC 20007

I certify that I served a copy of this pleading on July 28, 2011 by US mail to: Mary Kelly, Esq., Office of the Solicitor, USPTO,
PO Box 1450
Alexandria, Va. 22313-1450